Guideline of Oral Care in Hematopoietic Stem Cell Transplantation

The Japanese Society of Oral Care

Akira Arasaki, Akihide Negishi,
Kazuto Hoshi, Nagato Natsume

Guideline of Oral Care in Hematopoietic Stem Cell Transplantation

Edited by : The Japanese Society of Oral Care

Akira Arasaki, Akihide Negishi,
Kazuto Hoshi, Nagato Natsume

This book was originally published in Japanese under the title of:
Zouketsusaibouisyoku kanjya no koukukea gaidorain (Guideline of Oral Care in Hematopoietic Stem Cell Transplantation)
Natsume Nagato et al.
©2015 1st ed. Ippanzaidan Houjin Kouku Hoken Kyokai
1-43-9, Komagome, Toshima-ku,
Tokyo 170-0003, Japan

All rights reserved. This book or any part may not be reproduced, stored in a system, or transmitted in any form or any means, electric, mechanical, photocopying, recording, or otherwise without prior written permission from publisher.

Printed by NEOMEDIX CO., LTD
5-22-28 Chiyoda, Naka-ku Nagoya 460-0012, Japan
Tel:+81-052-241-7428
FAX:+81-052-241-7959

Edited and Sold by NAGASUESHOTEN., LTD
69-2 Itsutsujicho, Kamigyo-ku, Kyoto 602-8446, Japan
Tel:+81-075-415-7280
FAX:+81-075-415-7290
19 March 2025
ISBN 978-4-8160-1450-5 C3047 ¥1364

JSPS KAKENHI Grant Number 23HP6001

Preface

This book is an English translation of a Japanese text created by the "Guideline Creation Subcommittee for Oral Care of Hematopoietic Stem Cell Transplantation (HSCT) Patients" within the Academic Committee of the Japanese Society of Oral Care, with the support of the Ministry of Education, Culture, Sports, Science and Technology's Research Grant-in-Aid for Publication of Scientific Research Results.

Oral care has become a critical component of patient health management, particularly in the context of hematopoietic stem cell transplantation. The importance of professional oral care in these patients cannot be overstated, and the methods and effectiveness of such care continue to evolve rapidly. However, the provision of oral care involves a variety of healthcare professionals, and there have been reported issues such as medical accidents related to oral care or infections resulting from insufficient oral care. Therefore, it is essential for healthcare providers to not only understand the guidelines presented in this book but also to stay up-to-date with the latest knowledge and techniques in oral care and hematopoietic stem cell transplantation.

This book aims to serve as an essential guide for all professionals involved in the care of hematopoietic stem cell transplantation patients, helping to resolve these issues and provide safer, more effective oral care. It is not enough to merely understand the content presented here; healthcare providers must continuously seek out and incorporate the latest information into their practice to provide high-quality care and safeguard patient health and safety.

We would like to express our sincere gratitude to Mr. Nagato Natsume, President of the Japanese Society of Oral Care; Mr. Kazuto Hoshi, Vice President of the Society; Mr. Akihide Negishi, Chair of the Guideline Creation Committee; and Mr. Hideki Nagasue of Nagasue Shoten for their tremendous efforts in the publication of this book.

The Japanese Society of Oral Care

Akira Arasaki

Contents

Chapter 1 The Purpose of Oral Care for Hematopoietic Stem Cell Transplant Patients ·· 1

Chapter 2 Overview of Hematopoietic Stem Cell Transplantation and Epidemiology ································· 5

1. Overview of Hematopoietic Stem Cell Transplantation ································· 6

2. The Process of Allogeneic Hematopoietic Stem Cell Transplantation ··············· 7

3. The Process of Autologous Hematopoietic Stem Cell Transplantation ············· 11

Chapter 3 Oral Evaluation ································· 15

1. Initial Assessment ································· 16

2. Evaluation during Neutropenic Period from Preconditioning to Engraftment (10–30 Days Post-transplant) ································· 20

3. Evaluation during Engraftment and Hematopoietic Reconstitution (Up to 100 Days Post-transplant) ································· 26

4. Evaluation Post-Treatment (After 100 Days) ································· 27

Chapter 4　Oral Adverse Events ⋯⋯⋯⋯⋯⋯⋯⋯⋯⋯⋯⋯⋯⋯⋯⋯ 31

1. Oral Adverse Events Associated with Pre-Transplant Conditioning ⋯⋯⋯⋯ 32

2. Oral Adverse Events Associated with Acute GvHD ⋯⋯⋯⋯⋯⋯⋯⋯⋯ 35

3. Oral Adverse Events Associated with Chronic GvHD ⋯⋯⋯⋯⋯⋯⋯⋯ 36

Chapter 5　Prevention of Oral Adverse Events ⋯⋯⋯⋯⋯⋯⋯ 43

1. Preventive Strategies for Oral Adverse Events (Overview) ⋯⋯⋯⋯⋯⋯⋯ 44

2. Efficacy of Oral Care as Prevention of Oral Adverse Events ⋯⋯⋯⋯⋯ 46

3. Flow of Prevention Strategies for Oral Adverse Events ⋯⋯⋯⋯⋯⋯⋯ 48

4. Oral Hygiene Instruction ⋯⋯⋯⋯⋯⋯⋯⋯⋯⋯⋯⋯⋯⋯⋯⋯⋯⋯⋯ 50

5. Dental Treatment to Be Performed Before Transplantation ⋯⋯⋯⋯⋯⋯ 54

6. Cryotherapy ⋯⋯⋯⋯⋯⋯⋯⋯⋯⋯⋯⋯⋯⋯⋯⋯⋯⋯⋯⋯⋯⋯⋯ 59

7. Systemic Adverse Events such as Bacteremia and Sepsis ⋯⋯⋯⋯⋯⋯ 60

Chapter 6　Management of Oral Adverse Events ⋯⋯⋯⋯ 69

1. Oral Mucositis ⋯⋯⋯⋯⋯⋯⋯⋯⋯⋯⋯⋯⋯⋯⋯⋯⋯⋯⋯⋯ 70

2. Oral Bacterial Infections ⋯⋯⋯⋯⋯⋯⋯⋯⋯⋯⋯⋯⋯⋯⋯ 71

3. Oral Candidiasis ⋯⋯⋯⋯⋯⋯⋯⋯⋯⋯⋯⋯⋯⋯⋯⋯⋯⋯⋯ 72

4. Oral Bleeding ⋯⋯⋯⋯⋯⋯⋯⋯⋯⋯⋯⋯⋯⋯⋯⋯⋯⋯⋯⋯ 73

5. GvHD ⋯⋯⋯⋯⋯⋯⋯⋯⋯⋯⋯⋯⋯⋯⋯⋯⋯⋯⋯⋯⋯⋯⋯⋯ 74

6. Dry Mouth ⋯⋯⋯⋯⋯⋯⋯⋯⋯⋯⋯⋯⋯⋯⋯⋯⋯⋯⋯⋯⋯⋯ 75

Chapter 7　Follow-up Observation ⋯⋯⋯⋯⋯⋯⋯⋯⋯⋯ 79

1. The Need for Follow-up Observation in Managing Oral Adverse Events ⋯⋯⋯ 80

2. Follow-up Interval and Duration After Hematopoietic Stem Cell

Transplantation ⋯⋯⋯⋯⋯⋯⋯⋯⋯⋯⋯⋯⋯⋯⋯⋯⋯⋯⋯ 82

Chapter 8　Prevention and Treatment in Children ⋯⋯⋯ 89

1. Characteristics of Hematopoietic Stem Cell Transplantation in Children ⋯⋯⋯ 90

2. Oral Adverse Events in Children ⋯⋯⋯⋯⋯⋯⋯⋯⋯⋯⋯⋯ 90

3. Considerations and Precautions for Oral Examination in Children ⋯⋯⋯⋯ 92

4. Key Points for Oral Care Nursing in Children ⋯⋯⋯⋯⋯⋯⋯ 92

Materials 96

Index 100

Chapter 1

The Purpose of Oral Care
for Hematopoietic Stem Cell
Transplant Patients

Chapter 1 The Purpose of Oral Care for Hematopoietic Stem Cell Transplant Patients

The recognition of the deep connection between oral care and overall health began when Yoneyama et al.[1] reported in the Lancet in 1999 that oral care reduced the incidence of aspiration pneumonia in elderly individuals requiring nursing care. Following this, further reports demonstrated the effectiveness of oral care in preventing ventilator-associated pneumonia (VAP) [2,3], as well as its impact on reducing postoperative complication rates in patients with head and neck cancer[4,5] and esophageal cancer[6] who received pre-hospital oral care.

On the other hand, Sonin et al.[7] compared groups of hematopoietic stem cell transplant patients with and without oral mucosal disorders. They found that patients with oral mucosal disorders had an increase of about 5 million yen per person in hospital costs compared to those without such disorders. Mogi et al. reported that specialized oral care for hematopoietic stem cell transplant patients resulted in reductions in the duration of fever, frequency and dosage of morphine use for oral pain, and a shortening of the period of inability to eat[8].

Hematopoietic stem cell transplant patients are those suffering from blood cell cancers, such as leukemia[9]. Their treatment involves chemotherapy and radiation therapy, similar to that of patients with other organ cancers. However, unlike other cancer patients, hematopoietic stem cell transplant patients undergo intensive chemotherapy and total body irradiation[10] to eradicate the cancerous blood cells. Additionally, because normal blood cells from a donor must be transplanted after the destruction of the cancerous cells, immunosuppressive drugs are required, leading to severe immune system suppression.

Chemotherapy and radiation therapy cause dry mouth and oral mucosal disorders. The causes of oral mucosal disorders include direct damage to oral mucosal cells from chemotherapy and radiation therapy, as well as the production of free radicals. If oral care is neglected, the growth of oral bacteria can lead to severe oral mucosal damage, with the possibility that oral lesions can become sources of infection, leading to bacteremia and even sepsis.

Oral care includes not only the care provided by nurses in hospital wards and home care settings but also specialized oral care by dental hygienists. Specialized oral care is defined as technical procedures performed by healthcare professionals to manage oral health, prevent oral diseases and pneumonia, and maintain or improve quality of life (QOL). It involves oral hygiene management and rehabilitation in the oral area, with the goal of assisting patients in maintaining a fulfilling daily life both physically and mentally[10].

Cancer patients undergoing chemotherapy and radiation therapy often experience a reduction in salivation due to salivary gland damage, which increases the likelihood of developing dry mouth and oral mucosal disorders. The onset of oral mucosal disorders causes oral pain, impaired eating function, avoidance of speaking, and sleep disturbances. Gastrointestinal issues such as nausea and diarrhea are also common, but the effects on the gastrointestinal tract are not limited to the stomach and intestines; the oral mucosa is similarly damaged.

Hematopoietic stem cell transplant patients not only face chemotherapy and radiation therapy, but also, following the transplant, may develop extensive and severe oral mucosal disorders due to immunosuppressive drug administration. As discussed above, oral care is effective in reducing oral mucosal damage, preventing severe infections, and preventing a decline in QOL.

(Nobuo Mogi, Tokyo Metropolitan Cancer and Infection Diseases Center Komagome

Hospital,, Department of Dentistry and Oral and Maxillofacial Surgery)

Chapter 1 The Purpose of Oral Care for Hematopoietic Stem Cell Transplant Patients

References

1 Yoneyama T, Yoshida M, Matsui T, and Sasaki H: Oral care and pneumonia, Oral Care Working Group, Lancet, 354 (9177): 515, 1999.

2 Sekishima M, Yamada T, Imamura S, Tokorozawa H, Kinoshita T, Matsushima R: Consideration of preventive measures for ventilator-associated pneumonia (VAP), Koshin Emergency Intensive Care Research, 18(1) : 95-100, 2002.

3 Fukuya S: Ventilator-associated pneumonia (VAP) and oral care Evidence-based prevention of ventilator-associated pneumonia (VAP), nursing techniques, 49(6) : 503-505, 2003.

4 Onishi T, Taniguchi Y, Matsui M, Itoh M: Oral care for head and neck cancer patients, The Japanese Society for Hygiene, 2(1):180-181, 2007.

5 Suzuki M, Fujiwara K, Ogami M, Hayashi M, Yasutomi M, et al: Professional oral care efforts in head and neck radiotherapy, Department of Oral Medicine and Pharyngology, 19(1): 85, 2006.

6 Yoshida H, Ishitobi S, Nogami T, Ayuse T, Ooi K: Actual status of feeding and swallowing rehabilitation for esophageal cancer patients among party members, Dentistry for the Disabled, 30(3): 387, 2009.

7 Sonis ST, Oster G, Fuchs H, Bellm L, Bradford WZm et al: Oral mucositis and the clinical and economic outcomes of hematopoietic stem-cell transplantation, J Clin Oncol, 18(8): 2201-2205, 2001.

8 Mogi S, Ikegami Y, NaritaK, Minagawa H, Tsuji M, et al: Effect of oral care on hematopoietic cell transplant patients on length of hospital stay, official publication of the Japanese Society of Oral Care, 1(1): 14-20, 2007.

9 Mogi N: leukemia, Dental hygiene, 29(11): 1216-1217, 2009.

10 Ikegami Y, Narita K, Mogi N: Oral care during hematopoietic stem cell transplantation: High-dose chemotherapy in pre-transplant treatment with the aim of providing care linked to meals, Oral care for patients receiving whole body radiation, Japanese Journal of Cancer Nursing, 13(3): 387-391, 2008.

Chapter 2

Overview of Hematopoietic Stem Cell Transplantation and Epidemiology

Chapter 2　Overview of Hematopoietic Stem Cell Transplantation and Epidemiology

1. Overview of Hematopoietic Stem Cell Transplantation

Hematopoietic stem cell transplantation (HSCT) is performed with the goal of reconstructing the hematopoietic and immune systems by transplanting the patient's own or a donor's hematopoietic stem cells. HSCT is most often used to treat hematologic malignancies such as leukemia and malignant lymphoma, but can also be applied to benign blood disorders like aplastic anemia, autoimmune diseases, and congenital metabolic disorders. HSCT is broadly classified into two types: autologous HSCT (where the patient's own hematopoietic stem cells are transplanted) and allogeneic HSCT (where a donor's hematopoietic stem cells are transplanted).

Autologous transplantation is performed after intensive chemotherapy or radiation therapy when recovery of hematopoiesis is expected to be insufficient. Allogeneic transplantation is typically performed using a donor with a compatible human leukocyte antigen (HLA). In addition to hematopoietic recovery, allogeneic HSCT is often performed with the expectation of graft-versus-host immune effects. Since the discovery of the importance of HLA in the late 1960s, allogeneic bone marrow transplants became possible[1], and the first transplant in Japan was conducted in the early 1970s. In recent years, HSCT has diversified, and with the spread of reduced-intensity conditioning (RIC) and mini-transplants, even elderly patients and those with organ dysfunction can now undergo transplantation, making it possible to treat hematologic diseases more common in older adults, such as myelodysplastic syndrome[2].

Additionally, peripheral blood stem cells and umbilical cord blood are now used as alternative sources of hematopoietic stem cells[3]. Traditionally, allogeneic peripheral blood stem cell transplants could only be performed with related donors, but since 2010, they have also been possible with unrelated donors. Furthermore, transplants from HLA-incompatible donors have also been performed in a significant number of cases (Table 1).

6

Table 1 Classification of Hematopoietic Cell Transplantation

1. Autologous/Allogeneic Transplantation
    Autologous Transplantation
    Allogeneic Transplantation
    Classification by Transplanted Cells

2. Bone Marrow Transplantation
    Peripheral Blood Stem Cell Transplantation
    Umbilical Cord Blood Transplantation
    Classification by Pretransplantation Conditioning

3. Myeloablative Conditioning
    Non-Myeloablative Conditioning
    Classification by Donor

4. Related Donor
    Unrelated Donor
    HLA-Matched Donor
    HLA-Mismatched Donor

With the expansion of transplant methods and donor sources, the number of transplants performed annually has been increasing. In Japan, during the 2009 fiscal year, approximately 2,300 allogeneic transplants and 1,350 autologous transplants were performed[4].

2. The Process of Allogeneic Hematopoietic Stem Cell Transplantation

Most patients who undergo HSCT are those with hematologic malignancies, and many have a history of chemotherapy. Patients with benign hematologic diseases, such as aplastic anemia and immune disorders, are typically treated with immunosuppressive therapy and blood transfusion

Chapter 2 Overview of Hematopoietic Stem Cell Transplantation and Epidemiology

therapy. Since these patients may have developed conditions like oral mucositis and dry mouth during previous treatments, it is important to assess their treatment history and any complications before transplantation[5].

Pre-transplant conditioning is typically performed about one week before the transplantation. The goals of pre-transplant conditioning are (1) to suppress the patient's immune system to promote engraftment of the transplanted cells and (2) to provide antitumor effects. In the past, intensive chemotherapy and radiation therapy were used to achieve both goals, but due to regimen-related toxicities (RRT), this could not be applied to elderly patients or those with organ dysfunction. Recently, the focus has shifted toward immune suppression in non-myeloablative conditioning regimens, which has made transplantation possible for elderly patients, those with organ dysfunction, and those with a history of autologous transplantation. The intensity of pre-conditioning, the type of chemotherapy used, and the presence or absence of radiation affect the risk of oral mucositis.

After conditioning, hematopoietic stem cells are transplanted. Allogeneic transplantation is divided into three major phases:

Phase 1 (pre-engraftment): From pre-transplant conditioning to neutrophil engraftment.

Phase 2 (early post-engraftment): From engraftment to approximately day 100.

Phase 3 (late post-engraftment): From day 100 onwards.

Each phase requires management of specific complications (Figure. 1)[6]. In Phase 1, which spans from transplantation to neutrophil engraftment, blood cell counts decrease due to RRT, and mucosal damage such as oral mucositis and diarrhea persists for 2-4 weeks, making the patient highly susceptible to infections. During this period, patients are typically managed in a sterile room. Preventive treatments with acyclovir for herpes simplex virus, antifungal agents for Candida and Aspergillus, and broad-spectrum antibiotics, including quinolones, are common. Fever during neutropenia (febrile neutropenia, FN) is a major concern due to the high risk of

8

2. The Process of Allogeneic Hematopoietic Stem Cell Transplantation

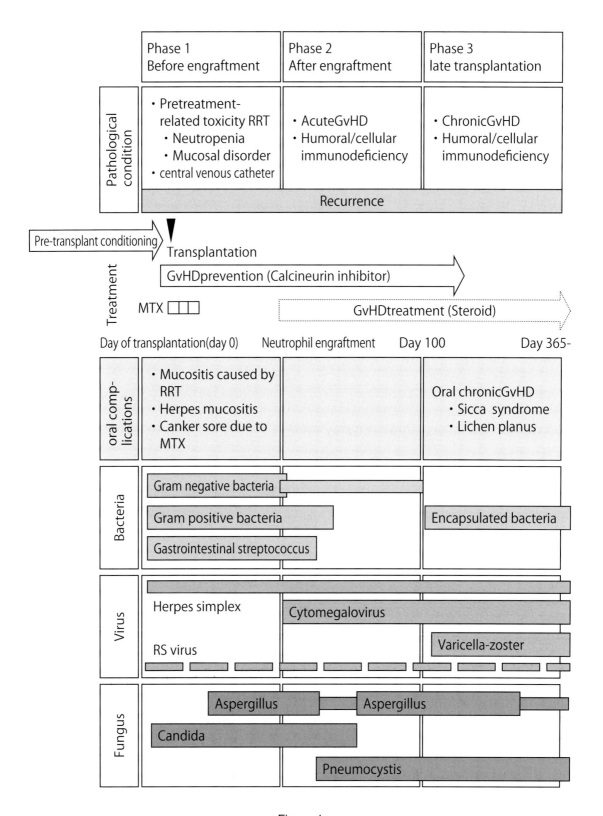

Figure 1

Chapter 2 Overview of Hematopoietic Stem Cell Transplantation and Epidemiology

severe infection, and broad-spectrum antibiotics are administered even before the causative organism is identified.

The time to neutrophil engraftment varies by stem cell source: 10-14 days for peripheral blood stem cell transplantation, 2-3 weeks for bone marrow transplantation, and 3-4 weeks for umbilical cord blood transplantation. Around 20% of umbilical cord blood transplantations experience engraftment failure[7]. As neutrophil recovery occurs, mucosal damage improves. Platelets typically recover 1-2 weeks after neutrophil recovery. Early post-transplant immunosuppressive drugs, such as cyclosporine or tacrolimus, are combined with methotrexate (MTX) and mycophenolate mofetil (MMF) to prevent graft-versus-host disease (GvHD). MTX is a known cause of oral mucositis before engraftment.

In Phase 2, from engraftment to day 100, management focuses on acute GvHD and infections related to immune deficiency[8]. GvHD is an immune reaction in which donor-derived immune cells attack the patient's organs, and it is classified into acute and chronic forms. Acute GvHD typically occurs within 100 days after transplantation and primarily affects the skin, gastrointestinal tract, and liver. Symptoms in these organs are assessed (staging) and the severity of acute GvHD is determined (grading). Severe cases may require steroid treatment. During this time, viral infections such as cytomegalovirus (CMV), as well as fungal infections like Aspergillus and Pneumocystis, are significant concerns. CMV is monitored regularly with PCR testing or antigenemia, and antiviral treatment is started upon reactivation to prevent pneumonia or enteritis. Pneumocystis infections are prevented with prophylactic trimethoprim-sulfamethoxazole (ST) therapy.

After day 100, chronic GvHD is generally defined, with symptoms in the skin, liver, and other organs, including dryness in the eyes and mouth, oral lichen planus, and respiratory symptoms. GvHD treatment with steroids may exacerbate post-transplant immunosuppression, increasing the risk of various infections. The management of these infections can be challenging, and chronic

GvHD often results in a significant decline in quality of life. Chronic GvHD and associated immunodeficiency are considered part of Phase 3.

For patients with hematologic malignancies, allogeneic HSCT is performed with the expectation of graft-versus-tumor (GvT) effects, although it is currently difficult to separate GvHD from GvT effects[9].

3. The Process of Autologous Hematopoietic Stem Cell Transplantation

Autologous transplantation is used to eradicate malignant tumors with intensive chemotherapy, followed by autologous stem cell transplantation to restore hematopoiesis. Typically, patients up to age 65-70 undergo autologous transplantation, and it is most often performed in patients with malignancies such as lymphoma and multiple myeloma. Some chemotherapy-sensitive solid tumors may also be treated with this method. The patient's hematopoietic stem cells are collected and cryopreserved during chemotherapy, and after intensive chemotherapy, these cells are transplanted to restore blood cell production.

In most cases, peripheral blood stem cells are used for autologous transplantation. The time to engraftment is typically 10-14 days, and engraftment failure is rare. The RRT during engraftment is similar to allogeneic transplantation, with mucosal damage and infection prevention required, but GvHD does not occur, so immunosuppressive drugs are not necessary. The risk of complications after engraftment is lower than in allogeneic transplantation, and the rate of complications-related mortality is less than 10%. However, unlike allogeneic transplantation, no GvT effect is expected, and the possibility of tumor cells contaminating the transplant cells cannot be ruled out, meaning the risk of relapse remains high.

Chapter 2 Overview of Hematopoietic Stem Cell Transplantation and Epidemiology

(Akio Shigematsu, Department of Laboratory Medicine and Transfusion, Hematopoietic Cell

Therapy Center, Hokkaido University Hospital)

References

1 Little MT and Storb R: History of hematopoietic stem cell transplantation, Nat Rev, Cancer, 2: 231-
238, 2002.

2 Servais S, Baron F and Beguin Y: Allogeneic hematopoietic stem cell transplantation (HSCT) after
reduced-intensity conditioning. Allogeneic hematopoietic stem cell transplantation (HSCT), Transfus
Apher Sci, 44(2): 205-210, 2011.

3 Gluckman E: A decade of cord blood transplantation, from bench to bedside, Br J Haematol, 147(2):
192-199, 2009.

4 The Japanese Society for Hematopoietic Cell Transplantation: 2010 National Survey Report, Japan
Society for Hematopoietic Cell Transplantation Datacenter, Nagoya 2011

5 Niscola P, Romani C, Cupelli L, et al: Mucositis in patients with hematologic malignancies an
overview, Haematologica, 92(2): 222-231, 2007.

6 Center for International Blood and Marrow Transplant Research (CIBMTR), National Marrow Donor
Program (NMDP), European Blood and Marrow Transplant Group (EBMT), American Society
for Blood and Marrow Transplantation (ASBMT), Canadian Blood and Marrow Transplant Group
(CBMTG), Infectious Diseases Society of America (IDSA), Society for Healthcare Epidemiology of
America (SHEA), Canadian Association for Medical Microbiology and Infection (AMMI), Centers for
Disease Control and Prevention (CDC): Guidelines for the prevention of infectious complications in
hematopoietic cell transplant recipients a global perspective, Bone Marrow Transplant, 44(8): 453-558,
2009.

7 Urbano-Ispizua A: Risk assessment in hematopoietic stem cell transplantation stem cell source, Best Pract Res Clin Haematol, 20(2): 265-280, 2007.

8 Hematopoietic cell transplantation guidelines gvhd, Japanese Society for Hematopoietic Cell Transplantation, http://www.jshct.com/guideline/pdf/2009gvhd.pdf.

9 Weiden PL, Sullivan KM, Flournoy N, et al: Antileukemic effect of chronic graft-versus-host disease contribution to improved survival after allogeneic marrow transplantation, N Engl J Med, 304: 1529-3153, 1981.

Chapter **3**

Oral Evaluation

Chapter 3 Oral Evaluation

1. Initial Assessment

Before initiating hematopoietic stem cell transplantation (HSCT), it is essential to understand the patient's disease type, previous treatments, and disease condition to evaluate their overall health status. Furthermore, in the case of full transplants, a high-dose chemotherapy regimen and total body irradiation are typically administered as preparatory treatments to eradicate both cancer and bone marrow cells. This leads to the expectation of more adverse events than those typically seen in regular radiation therapy or chemotherapy.

Before beginning oral procedures, a comprehensive assessment of the underlying disease and organ dysfunction is necessary to ensure appropriate measures are taken. Following this, an evaluation of the oral cavity and teeth should be conducted to perform treatments before the transplant and to reduce potential oral complications after the transplant through proper oral care[1-13].

1) General Assessment

When conducting oral evaluations and treatments, it is necessary to gather information on the underlying disease and organ dysfunctions[14].

(1) Assessment of underlying disease: Disease type, condition, previous treatments, and remission induction protocols.

(2) Assessment related to transplantation: Type of transplant and medications to be administered.

(3) Evaluation of other organ dysfunctions: Cardiovascular, respiratory, liver function, renal function, infections, and allergies.

16

2) Oral Evaluation

Caries and periodontal disease can become severe infection foci after transplantation, so it is crucial to treat them as much as possible before the procedure. Additionally, oral care can help reduce mucosal damage. Oral and dental assessments should be conducted before transplantation, followed by appropriate management and guidance[15]. The Eilers J. Oral Assessment Criteria, which is the standard in the U.S., can also be a helpful tool for evaluation (Table 2)[16].

(1) Dental treatment history: Confirm past treatments through a questionnaire, oral examination, and X-rays. Evaluate whether restorative or prosthetic devices could cause mucosal damage, if there are any bridges hindering brushing, and the success of endodontic treatments.

(2) Symptomatic teeth: Evaluate symptomatic teeth, including pain and swelling, and confirm the type, severity, and onset time of symptoms as well as whether treatment has been performed. Treatment planning should take the timing of transplantation into account.

(3) History of trauma: Assess whether there is a history of jawbone fractures, including the site, severity, treatment, and healing status. Evaluate whether any problems related to fixed appliances, deformed healing, or malocclusion have emerged.

(4) History of radiation therapy: If there is a history of radiation therapy to the oral and maxillofacial area, invasive treatments like tooth extractions may be restricted.

(5) Oral habits: Habits like bruxism, tooth contacting, or tongue thrusting may contribute to mucosal damage or temporomandibular joint disorders.

(6) Previous care, prevention methods, and adherence: Review the oral care and dental disease prevention methods the patient has received previously, along with adherence to them. Confirm ongoing management by the dentist or dental hygienist and continue as needed.

Chapter 3　Oral Evaluation

(7) Oral hygiene status: Assess plaque scores, tongue coating, and mucosal contamination, and create an appropriate care plan.

(8) Radiological evaluation: Evaluate alveolar bone resorption, periapical lesions, impacted teeth, and intraosseous lesions to determine if periodontal treatment, endodontic therapy, tooth extraction, or surgical intervention is necessary[17].

3) Prioritization of Dental Procedures

Ideally, all dental treatments should be completed before initiating transplant therapy. To achieve this, patients should be referred to a dentist as early as possible when transplantation is scheduled to ensure sufficient time for treatment. The priority should be to eliminate infection foci and address potential symptoms or mucosal damage[5,8,10].

(1) Treatment for infection foci: Root canal therapy should be completed at least one week before the pre-transplant conditioning if possible. If not feasible, tooth extraction may be necessary[10].

(2) Tooth extraction: Extraction should be considered for broken teeth, carious teeth with acute symptoms, impacted teeth, periodontal disease-affected teeth with significant bone resorption or furcation lesions, or wisdom teeth with suspected inflammation. These procedures should be completed at least two weeks before the pre-transplant conditioning[1,5,8,10,11].

(3) Periodontal disease treatment and management: Scaling, preventive treatments, and brushing instruction should be provided[5,10].

(4) Removal of mucosal irritants: Sharp-edged teeth, restorative materials, crowns, dentures, or orthodontic devices that may cause mucosal damage should be adjusted or removed.

(5) Carious teeth that may cause pulp infection or pain: Treatment should be carried out within a reasonable time frame, considering the treatment period.

1. Initial Assessment

Table 2 Eilers J.'s Oral Assessment Index[16].

Category	Tools for Assessment	Methods of Measurement	Score1	Score2	Score3
Voice	Auditory assessment	Converse with patient	Normal	Deeper or raspy	Difficulty talking or painful
Swallow	Observation	Ask patient to swallow. To test gag reflex, gently place blade on back of tongue and depress	Normal swallow	Some pain on swallow	Unable to swallow
Lips	Visual/ palpatory	Observe and feel tissue	Smooth and pink and moist	Dry or cracked	Ulcerated or bleeding
Tongue	Visual/ palpatory	Feel and observe appearance of tissue	Pink and moist and papillae present	Coated or loss of papillae with shiny appearance with or without redness	Blistered or cracked
Saliva	Tongue blade	Insert blade into mouth, touching the center of the tongue and the floor of the mouth	Watery	Thick or ropy	Absent
Mucous membranes	Visual assessment	Observe appearance of tissue	Pink and moist	Reddened or coated (increased whiteness) without ulcerations	Ulcerations with or without bleeding
Gingiva	Tongue blade and visual assessment	Gently press tissue with tip of blade	Pink and stippled and firm	Edematous with or without redness	Spontaneous bleeding or bleeding with pressure
Teeth, Dentures, or denture bearing area	Visual assessment	Observe appearance of teeth or denture bearing area	Clean and no debris	Plaque or debris in localized areas (between teeth if present)	Plaque or debris generalized along gum line or denture bearing area

19

Chapter 3 Oral Evaluation

2. Evaluation during Neutropenic Period from Preconditioning to Engraftment (10–30 Days Post-transplant)

During the preconditioning phase of hematopoietic stem cell transplantation, intensive chemotherapy and total body irradiation often lead to neutropenia, causing adverse events like oral mucositis and dry mouth. Oral health should be closely monitored to manage these adverse events effectively.

1) Oral Evaluation

Adverse events common in cancer patients are evaluated using the Common Terminology Criteria for Adverse Events (CTCAE), which is internationally recognized and published by the U.S. National Cancer Institute (NCI). The latest version is the 4th edition, and the Japanese translation is available through the Japan Clinical Oncology Group (JCOG) on their website[18]. The evaluation criteria for oral adverse events are listed in each section. The Eilers J. Oral Assessment Criteria (Table 2) can also be applied for evaluation.

(1) Oral hygiene status: Assess plaque accumulation, tongue coating, and mucosal contamination. When providing oral hygiene guidance, consider platelet counts (<40,000, 40,000–75,000, 75,000<) when determining brushing methods and tools[1-12].

2. Evaluation during Neutropenic Period from Preconditioning to Engraftment (10–30 Days Post-transplant)

(2) Oral mucositis: Assess the affected area, presence of bleeding, and pain severity. Consider the cause of mucosal irritation and pain relief methods. Nutritional status should also be evaluated[5-11,19].

	Grade 1	Grade 2	Grade 3	Grade 4	Grade 5
Mucositis oral	Asymptomatic or mild symptoms; intervention not indicated	Moderate pain or ulcer that does not interfere with oral intake; modified diet indicated	Severe pain; interfering with oral intake	Life-threatening consequences; urgent intervention indicated	Death
Cheilitis	Asymptomatic; clinical or diagnostic observations only; intervention not indicated	Moderate symptoms; limiting instrumental ADL	Severe symptoms; limiting self care ADL; intervention indicated	-	-

21

Chapter 3　Oral Evaluation

(3) Oral mucosal infections: Determine the causative organism (fungal, viral, bacterial) to
guide treatment[1,5,8-11].

	Grade 1	Grade 2	Grade 3	Grade 4	Grade 5
Mucosal infection	Localized, local intervention indicated	Oral intervention indicated (e.g., antibiotic, antifungal, or antiviral)	IV antibiotic, antifungal, or antiviral intervention indicated; invasive intervention indicated	Life-threatening consequences; urgent intervention indicated	Death
Lip infection	Localized, local intervention indicated	Oral intervention indicated (e.g., antibiotic, antifungal, or antiviral)	IV antibiotic, antifungal, or antiviral intervention indicated; invasive intervention indicated	-	-
Gum infection	Local therapy indicated (swish and swallow)	Moderate symptoms; oral intervention indicated (e.g., antibiotic, antifungal, or antiviral)	IV antibiotic, antifungal, or antiviral intervention indicated; invasive intervention indicated	Life-threatening consequences; urgent intervention indicated	Death

2. Evaluation during Neutropenic Period from Preconditioning to Engraftment (10–30 Days Post-transplant)

(4) Oral bleeding

	Grade 1	Grade 2	Grade 3	Grade 4	Grade 5
Oral hemorrhage	Mild symptoms; intervention not indicated	Moderate symptoms; intervention indicated	Transfusion indicated; invasive intervention indicated; hospitalization	Life-threatening consequences; urgent intervention indicated	Death

(5) Oral pain

	Grade 1	Grade 2	Grade 3	Grade 4	Grade 5
Oral pain	Mild pain	Moderate pain; limiting instrumental ADL	Severe pain; limiting self care ADL	-	-
Lip pain	Mild pain	Moderate pain; limiting instrumental ADL	Severe pain; limiting self care ADL	-	-
Gingival pain	Mild pain	Moderate pain interfering with oral intake	Severe pain; inability to aliment orally	-	-

Chapter 3 Oral Evaluation

(6) Tooth hypersensitivity/pain: This may occur when alkaloid chemotherapy agents are

administered. Typical treatments for hypersensitivity may not be effective[5-8,10].

	Grade 1	Grade 2	Grade 3	Grade 4	Grade 5
Toothache	Mild pain	Moderate pain; limiting instrumental ADL	Severe pain; limiting self care ADL	-	-

(7) Oral dryness: Evaluate the severity of dryness and consider appropriate moisturizing

treatments[8,20].

	Grade 1	Grade 2	Grade 3	Grade 4	Grade 5
Dry mouth	Symptomatic (e.g., dry or thick saliva) without significant dietary alteration; unstimulated saliva flow > 0.2 ml/min	Moderate symptoms; oral intake alterations (e.g., copious water, other lubricants, diet limited to purees and/or soft, moist foods); unstimulated saliva 0.1 to 0.2 ml/min	Inability to adequately aliment orally; tube feeding or TPN indicated; unstimulated saliva < 0.1 ml/min	-	-

(8) Trismus: Assess whether opening exercises are needed and when to start them[3,5-10].

	Grade 1	Grade 2	Grade 3	Grade 4	Grade 5
Trismus	Decreased ROM (range of motion) without impaired eating	Decreased ROM requiring small bites, soft foods or purees	Decreased ROM with inability to adequately aliment or hydrate orally	-	-

(9) Dysgeusia

	Grade 1	Grade 2	Grade 3	Grade 4	Grade 5
Dysgeusia	Altered taste but no change in diet	Altered taste with change in diet (e.g., oral supplements); noxious or unpleasant taste; loss of taste	-	-	-

2) Frequency of Observation and Evaluation

Oral mucositis, dry mouth, oral pain, oral bleeding, opportunistic infections, and dysgeusia may appear due to chemotherapy, radiation therapy, and supportive treatments. Frequent observation and evaluation should be conducted at least once a day to address oral changes and implement appropriate management. While proper oral care is essential, dental treatments should be avoided, and supportive therapies should be considered for acute symptoms[15].

Chapter 3 Oral Evaluation

3. Evaluation during Engraftment and Hematopoietic Reconstitution (Up to 100 Days Post-transplant)

Oral adverse events related to chemotherapy, radiation therapy, and supportive care begin to decrease as engraftment and hematopoietic reconstitution take place around 3–4 weeks post-transplant. However, this period may also see the onset of acute GvHD and viral infections.

1) Oral Evaluation

(1) Oral hygiene status: Assess plaque accumulation, tongue coating, and mucosal contamination, and consider appropriate hygiene management methods[1-11].

(2) Fungal and viral infections

(3) Tooth hypersensitivity/pain

(4) Oral dryness

(5) Oral GvHD: Symptoms such as erosion and blister formation are similar to mucositis. Differentiating between oral GvHD and mucosal damage caused by chemotherapy or radiation therapy can be difficult. When oral GvHD occurs, other organs such as the skin, liver, and gastrointestinal tract may also be affected[5,8].

2) Frequency of Observation and Evaluation

Adverse events begin to decrease around 3–4 weeks after transplantation. Oral mucositis, dry mouth, oral ulcers, and oral GvHD may develop. Daily oral examinations and at least weekly evaluations should be conducted, considering oral hygiene, dry mouth, mucositis, and oral GvHD management. Acute GvHD is primarily characterized by skin, liver, and gastrointestinal damage, requiring treatment with immunosuppressants, which necessitates coordination with the primary physician. Invasive dental treatments should be evaluated in collaboration with the primary physician due to the sustained immunosuppressive state[15].

4. Evaluation Post-Treatment (After 100 Days)

After 100 days post-transplantation, immune function is reconstituted, and chronic toxicities associated with maintenance therapy can result in oral adverse events. Late viral infections, chronic oral GvHD, and developmental abnormalities in children (such as dental and craniofacial growth issues) may occur.

1) Oral Evaluation

(1) Oral hygiene status: Evaluate whether optimal oral hygiene is maintained[1-11].

(2) Late viral infections: Be aware of oral mucosal symptoms related to herpes simplex or papillomavirus infections[8].

(3) Chronic oral GvHD: Symptoms such as lichen planus-like changes, leukoplakia-like changes, or sclerotic lesions that cause opening difficulties are early signs of chronic GvHD. Leukoplakia can transition to secondary cancer (squamous cell carcinoma), so regular monitoring and biopsies are recommended. It is necessary to differentiate chronic GvHD from infections caused by viruses or fungi and lesions treated with local steroids. Chronic GvHD may present with symptoms such as dry mouth, mucosal atrophy, mucous cysts, pseudo membranes, and ulcer formation. If other diseases are ruled out through histological and imaging evaluations, chronic GvHD can be diagnosed[5,8].

(4) Salivary secretion issues and dry mouth: Evaluate the cause of symptoms, whether related to chronic GvHD or chemotherapy and radiation therapy. Consider the use of salivary stimulants or moisturizers[20].

Chapter 3 Oral Evaluation

(5) Osteomyelitis or necrosis of the jawbone: This can occur in patients who have undergone radiation therapy to the jaw or are using bisphosphonates. Assess for swelling, pain, bone exposure, or pus drainage[21].

(6) Trismus: This may be due to sclerotic changes in the oral mucosa from chronic GvHD or the effects of radiation therapy. Evaluate the cause and determine the appropriate time to begin opening exercises and pain management[3,5,10].

(7) Dental or craniofacial developmental abnormalities (in children): These may result from chemotherapy or radiation therapy, and the timing of the treatment will affect the manifestation of dental defects, formation abnormalities, and malocclusions. Treatment planning should consider the status of the underlying disease[21,22].

2) Frequency of Observation and Evaluation

Adverse events post-treatment requires long-term monitoring. In particular, chronic GvHD, secondary cancer, dry mouth, and craniofacial developmental abnormalities require appropriate treatment.

Oral hygiene and periodontal health should be evaluated at least every six months. If chronic GvHD, dry mouth, or trismus is present, more frequent evaluations (every 1–3 months) are needed, with interventions as necessary. For patients with immune deficiencies, invasive dental treatments should be avoided. Chronic GvHD can transition to secondary cancer, and craniofacial growth abnormalities may develop over a long period, requiring lifelong monitoring. Maintaining optimal oral health through proper evaluation and management is crucial.

(Akihide Negishi, Yokohama Medival Center, Department of Dentistry and Oral and

Maxillofacial Surgery)

References

1 Barker GJ: Current practices in the oral management of the patient undergoing chemotherapy or bone marrow transplantation, Support Care Cancer, 7(l): 17-20, 1999.

2 Sonis S, Kunz A: Impact of improved dental services on the frequency of oral complications of cancer therapy for patients with non-head-and-neck malignancies, Oral Surg Oral Med Oral Pathol, 65(l): 19-22, 1988.

3 Scully C, Epstein JB: Oral health care for the cancer patient, EurJ Cancer B Oral Oncol, 32B(5): 281-292, 1996.

4 Toth BB, Martin JW, Fleming TJ: Oral and dental care associated with cancer therapy, Cancer Bull, 43: 397-402, 1991.

5 Schubert MM, Epstein JB, Peterson DE: Oral complications of cancer therapy Pharmacology and Therapeutics for Dentistry, 5th ed, Mosby-Year Book Inc, St. Louis Mo, 797-813, 2004.

6 National Institutes of Health, National Cancer Institute: Consensus Development Conference on Oral Complications of Cancer Therapies Diagnosis Prevention and Treatment, National Cancer Institute Monograph, No. 9, Bethesda Md, National Institutes of Health, 1990.

7 Epstein JB, Schubert MM: Oral mucositis in myelosuppressive cancer therapy, Oral Surg Oral Med Oral Pathol Oral Radiol Endod, 88(3): 273-276, 1999.

8 Schubert MM, Peterson DE, Lloid ME: Oral complications. Thomas' Hematopoietic Cell Transplantation, 3rd ed, Blackwell Science Inc, Mass, 911-928, 2004.

9 Bavier AR: Nursing management of acute oral complications of cancer Consensus Development Conference on Oral Complications of Cancer Therapies Diagnosis Prevention and Treatment, National Cancer Institute Monograph No. 9, National Institutes of Health, Bethesda Md, 123-128, 1990.

10 Little JW, Falace DA, Miller CS, Rhodus NL: Dental Management of the Medically Compromised Patient, 7th ed, Mosby, St Louis Mo, 433-461, 2008.

11 Sonis S, Fazio RC, Fang L: Principles and Practice of Oral Medicine, 2nd ed, WB Saunders Co, Philadelphia Pa, 426-454, 1995.

12 Borowski B, Benhamou E, Pico JL, Laplanche A, Margainaud JP, Hayat M: Prevention of oral

mucositis in patients treated with high-dose chemotherapy and bone marrow transplantation A randomised controlled trial comparing two protocols of dental care, EurJ Cancer B Oral Oncol, 30B(2): 93-97, 1994.

13   Da Fonseea MA: Dental care of the pédiatrie cancer patient, Pediatr Dent, 26(l): 53-57, 2004.

14   Sorror ML, Maris MB, Storb R, Baron F, Sandmaier BM, Maloney DG, Storer B: Hematopoietic cell transplantation (HCT) -specific comorbidity index a new tool for risk assessment before allogeneic HCT, Blood, 106(8): 2912-2919, 2005.

15   American Academy on Pediatric Dentistry: Guideline on dental management of pediatric patients receiving chemotherapy hematopoietic cell transplantation, and/or radiation, Pediatr Dent, 30 (7 Suppl): 219-225, 2008-2009.

16   Eilers J, Berger AM, PEtersen MC: Developmet testing and application of the oral assessment guide, Oncol Nurs Forum, 15(3): 325-330, 1988.

17   Peters E, Monopoli M, Woo SB, Sonis S: Assessment of the need for treatment of postendodontic asymptomatic periapical radiolucencies in bone marrow transplant recipients, Oral Surg Oral Med Oral Pathol, 76(l): 45-48, 1993.

18   Japanese Clinical Oncology Research Group, Common Terminology Criteria for Adverse Events v4.0 Japanese translation JCOG version, http://www.jcog.jp/doctor/tool/CTCAEv4J_20111217.pdf.

19   Soga Y, Sugiura Y, Takahashi K, Nishimoto H, Maeda Y, Tanimoto M, Takashiba S: Progress of oral care and reduction of oral mucositis–a pilot study in a hematopoietic stem cell transplamtation ward, Support Care Cancer, 19(2): 303-307, 2011.

20   Nieuw Amerongen AV, Veerman ECI: Current therapies for xerostomia and salivary gland hypofunction associated with cancer therapies, Support Care Cancer, 11(4): 226-231, 2003.

21   Zahrowski JJ: Bisphosphonate treatment An orthodontic concern for a proactive approach, Am J Orthod Dentofacial Orthop, 131(3): 311-320, 2007.

22   Dahllöf G, Jonsson A, Ulmner M, Huggare J: Orrhodontic treatment in long-term survivors after bone marrow transplantation, Am J Orthod Dentof Orthop, 120(5): 459-465, 2001.

Chapter **4**

Oral Adverse Events

Chapter 4 Oral Adverse Events

1. Oral Adverse Events Associated with Pre-Transplant Conditioning

Oral adverse events in hematopoietic stem cell transplant (HSCT) patients vary depending on the conditioning regimen. These include mucositis, infections, oral bleeding, reduced salivation with oral infections, and taste alterations. The incidence of oral mucositis induced by chemotherapy is 30-40% in typical chemotherapy use, 70-90% during HSCT (high-dose chemotherapy), and nearly 100% when chemotherapy is combined with radiotherapy to the head and neck[1-5]. Oral mucositis can lead to severe progressive complications, making appropriate management crucial (Tables 3, 4)[6-11].

Table 3 Main anticancer drugs and adverse events used in standard conditioning regimen treatment

Classification	Common name	Product name	Adverse event
Alkylating agent	Cyclophosphamide	Endoxan	Bone marrow suppression, nausea, hair loss, hemorrhagic cystitis
Alkylating agent	Busulfex	Mabrin	Convulsions, bone marrow suppression, nausea, interstitial pneumonia
Alkylating agent	Melphalan	Alkeran	Infectious diseases, nausea, liver damage, bone marrow suppression
Alkylating agent	CBDCA	Paraplatin	Bone marrow suppression, interstitial pneumonia
Antimetabolite	Fludarabine	Furdala	Bone marrow suppression, vomiting, interstitial pneumonia, neuropsychiatric disorders, gastrointestinal bleeding
Topoisomerase inhibitor	VP-16	Pepcid	Bone marrow suppression/interstitial pneumonia

32

Table 4 Adverse events of radiation exposure

	Adverse events
Totalbody irradiation	Headache, nausea, dry mouth, oral mucositis, taste disorder, interstitial pneumonia, cataract

1) Mucositis

Mucositis ranges from mild inflammation to ulcerative mucosal damage. In patients undergoing hematopoietic stem cell transplants involving bone marrow destruction, common sites for mucositis are the edges of the tongue, buccal mucosa, and the inner lips. Mucositis typically peaks between days 6-12 post-transplant and resolves by days 14-18. It causes pain and swallowing difficulties, affecting the intake of food and oral medications, making it a major source of discomfort for these patients[6,12].

2) Infections

Oral mucositis in HSCT patients is prone to infections due to reduced immune function and impaired salivary gland function. Furthermore, prolonged neutropenia can lead to bacteremia or sepsis due to oral bacteria[13]. During chemotherapy-induced bone marrow suppression, acute infections such as periapical periodontitis and periodontal disease may occur[14-17], and the incidence of oral bacterial infections during chemotherapy has been reported as 5.8%[17]. Proper oral care before conditioning can significantly reduce the risk of infections and associated complications[18-20].

Chapter 4 Oral Adverse Events

3) Oral Bleeding

Oral bleeding occurs during the period of thrombocytopenia resulting from bone marrow suppression. When platelet counts fall below 10,000/μL, the risk of spontaneous oral bleeding significantly increases. In areas where mucositis has caused ulcers, submucosal vessels may be damaged, leading to bleeding. Similarly, gingivitis can cause gum bleeding[21].

4) Xerostomia

Xerostomia is caused by reduced salivary gland function. In HSCT patients, total body irradiation and chemotherapy during conditioning often impair salivary gland function[22], leading to an increased risk of xerostomia. Consequences of reduced salivary function include: loss of lubrication in the mouth, making mucosal damage more likely; decreased self-cleaning ability, leading to plaque buildup; impaired buffering capacity and pH, increasing the risk of caries; and heightened pathogenicity of the oral microbiota.

5) Taste Alterations

Patients undergoing allogeneic HSCT often experience changes or a reduction in their sense of taste. Calcineurin inhibitors such as cyclosporine (CSP) and tacrolimus (TAC) may cause metallic taste, altered perceptions of spicy, sweet, sour, and bitter flavors, or even complete loss of taste[23]. Dysgeusia typically last for several months but usually recover. These changes can lead to nausea, decreased food intake, and weight loss, significantly impacting quality of life.

2. Oral Adverse Events Associated with Acute GvHD

Oral adverse events change with the progression of acute graft-versus-host disease (GvHD). These events occur concurrently with the bone marrow suppression phase. Both infections and acute GvHD manifest simultaneously, and the rapidly dividing oral mucosa is susceptible to damage, leading to oral pain[24].

1) Symptoms

These may include erythema, atrophy, edema, and ulceration[25,26]. Eventually, these symptoms can spread throughout the oral mucosa, including the buccal mucosa and lips.

2) Causes

These events are caused by both acute GvHD and high-dose chemotherapy or radiotherapy, making it difficult to differentiate the origin of symptoms during this period.

3) Incidence

Oral adverse events are observed in 35-60% of transplant patients. They may appear as early as 1-2 weeks post-transplant, often occurring between days 18 and 100[27,28]. After engraftment, 89% of patients experience oral symptoms, with the most severe symptoms typically occurring from engraftment to 3 months, suggesting that oral symptoms of acute GvHD are most severe during this period[29].

Chapter 4 Oral Adverse Events

3. Oral Adverse Events Associated with Chronic GvHD

1) Mucositis

(1) Symptoms

Oral mucositis, atrophy, pseudomembranous ulcers, mucoceles, fibrosis around the mouth, xerostomia resembling Sjögren's syndrome, and lichen planus can all occur as oral mucosal symptoms. Oral ulcers are often covered with grayish or yellowish pseudomembrane-like clots[30-32]. The oral mucosa may show erythema, atrophy, disappearance of the stratum corneum, and loss of filiform papillae on the tongue, with erosions resembling tooth impressions appearing on the buccal mucosa and around the tongue. The attached gingiva around the upper anterior teeth shows atrophy, with a loss of stippling and moderate to severe inflammation[33]. In patients with chronic mucositis, vasculitis and capillary dilation may be present. Sclerotic changes around the mouth contribute to restricted mouth opening[34,35]. Additionally, reduced salivation leads to xerostomia and dysgeusia. Xerostomia increases the risk of caries, oral mucosal infections, pain, fragility, and difficulties with speech, chewing, and swallowing[36].

(2) Incidence

Reports from overseas indicate that oral mucositis is seen in 70% of peripheral blood stem cell transplants, 55% of bone marrow stem cell transplants, 33% of HLA-matched sibling bone marrow transplants, 49% of HLA-mismatched sibling bone marrow transplants, and 64% of HLA-matched unrelated bone marrow transplants[37]. In Japan, oral mucositis is reported in 35-48% of HLA-matched sibling bone marrow transplants and 45-77% of HLA-matched unrelated bone marrow transplants[38]. Among systemic symptoms of chronic GvHD, oral symptoms are the most frequent in bone marrow stem cell transplants and the second most frequent in peripheral blood stem cell transplants.

36

2) Dysgeusia

Dysgeusia can occur due to salivary gland dysfunction leading to xerostomia[39]. Oral candidiasis may also contribute to taste changes.

3) Oral Candidiasis

During steroid treatment, candidiasis can appear, particularly atrophic or erythematous forms, which are often associated with oral mucosal pain[40].

4) Secondary Cancer

In both adults and children with long-term survival, secondary cancers such as oral cancer, particularly squamous cell carcinoma and salivary gland tumors, can occur. The incidence of secondary cancers is reported to be 4-5 times higher than in the general population, with oral cancer incidence being more than 10 times higher[41-44].

(Nobuo Mogi et al, Tokyo Metropolitan Cancer and Infection Diseases Center Komagome Hospital,, Department of Dentistry and Oral and Maxillofacial Surgery)

References

1 Pico JL, Avila-Garavito A, Naccache P: Mucositis Its Occurrence Consequences and Treatment in the Oncology Setting, The oncologist, 3(6): 446-451, 1998.

2 McGuire DB, Altomonte V, Peterson DE, Wingard JR, Jones RJ, Grochow LB: Patterns of mucositis and pain in patients receiving preparative chemotherapy and bone marrow transplantation, Oncology nursing forum, 20(10): 1493-1502, 1993.

3 Woo SB, Sonis ST, Monopoli MM, Sonis AL: A longitudinal study of oral ulcerative mucositis in bone marrow transplant recipients, Cancer, 72(5): 1612-1617, 1993.

4 Carl W, Higby DJ: Oral manifestations of bone marrow transplantation, American journal of clinical oncology, 8(1): 81-87, 1985.

5 Naidu MU, Ramana GV, Rani PU, Mohan IK, Suman A, Roy P: Chemotherapy-induced and/or radiation therapy-induced oral mucositis-complicating the treatment of cancer, Neoplasia (New York, NY), 6(5): 423-431, 2004.

6 Sonis ST, Oster G, Fuchs H, Bellm L, Bradford WZ, Edelsberg J, et al: Oral mucositis and the clinical and economic outcomes of hematopoietic stem-cell transplantation, J Clin Oncol, 19(8): 2201-2205, 2001.

7 Elting LS, Cooksley C, Chambers M, Cantor SB, Manzullo E, Rubenstein EB: The burdens of cancer therapy, Clinical and economic outcomes of chemotherapy-induced mucositis, Cancer, 98(7): 1531-1539, 2003.

8 Elting LS, Cooksley CD, Chambers MS, Garden AS: Risk outcomes and costs of radiation-induced oral mucositis among patients with head-and-neck malignancies, International journal of radiation oncology biology physics, 68(4): 1110-1120, 2007.

9 Lalla RV, Sonis ST, Peterson DE: Management of oral mucositis in patients who have cancer, Dental clinics of North America, 52(1): 61-77, 2008.

10 Peterson DE, Lalla RV: Oral mucositis the new paradigms, Current opinion in oncology, 22(4): 318-322, 2010.

11 Rosenthal DI: Consequences of mucositis-induced treatment breaks and dose reductions on head and neck cancer treatment outcomes, The journal of supportive oncology, 5(9 Suppl 4): 23-31, 2007.

12 Elting LS, Avritscher EB, Cooksley CD, Cardenas-Turanzas M, Garden AS, Chambers MS: Psychosocial and economic impact of cancer, Dental clinics of North America, 52(1): 231-252, 2008.

13 Kennedy HF, Morrison D, Kaufmann ME, Jackson MS, Bagg J, Gibson BE, et al: Origins of Staphylococcus epidermidis and Streptococcus oralis causing bacteraemia in a bone marrow transplant patient, Journal of medical microbiology, 49(4): 367-370, 2000.

14 Graber CJ, de Almeida KN, Atkinson JC, Javaheri D, Fukuda CD, Gill VJ, et al: Dental health and viridans streptococcal bacteremia in allogeneic hematopoietic stem cell transplant recipients, Bone marrow transplantation, 27(5): 537-542, 2001.

15 Peterson DE, Minah GE, Overholser CD, Suzuki JB, DePaola LG, Stansbury DM, et al: Microbiology of acute periodontal infection in myelosuppressed cancer patients, J Clin Oncol, 5(9): 1461-1468, 1987.

16 Akintoye SO, Brennan MT, Graber CJ, McKinney BE, Rams TE, Barrett AJ, et al: A retrospective investigation of advanced periodontal disease as a risk factor for septicemia in hematopoietic stem cell and bone marrow transplant recipients, Oral surgery oral medicine oral pathology oral radiology and endodontics, 94(5): 581-588, 2002.

17 Hong CH, Napenas JJ, Hodgson BD, Stokman MA, Mathers-Stauffer V, Elting LS, et al: A systematic review of dental disease in patients undergoing cancer therapy, Support Care Cancer, 18(8): 1007-1021, 2010.

18 Peterson DE: Pretreatment strategies for infection prevention in chemotherapy patients, NCI Monogr, (9): 61-71, 1990.

19 Sonis ST, Woods PD, White BA: Oral complications of cancer therapies, retreatment oral assessment, NCI Monogr, (9): 29-32, 1990.

20 Peters E, Monopoli M, Woo SB, Sonis S: Assessment of the need for treatment of postendodontic asymptomatic periapical radiolucencies in bone marrow transplant recipients, Oral surgery oral medicine and oral pathology, 76(1): 45-8, 1993.

21 Wandt H, Frank M, Ehninger G, Schneider C, Brack N, Daoud A, et al: Safety and cost effectiveness of a 10 x 10^9/L trigger for prophylactic platelet transfusions compared with the traditional 20 x 10^9/L trigger a prospective comparative trial in 105 patients with acute myeloid leukemia, Blood, 91(10): 3601-3606, 1998.

Chapter 4 Oral Adverse Events

22 Jensen SB, Pedersen AM, Vissink A, Andersen E, Brown CG, Davies AN, et al: A systematic review of salivary gland hypofunction and xerostomia induced by cancer therapies prevalence severity and impact on quality of life, Support Care Cancer, 18(8): 1039-1060, 2010.

23 Marinone MG, Rizzoni D, Ferremi P, Rossi G, Izzi T, Brusotti C: Late taste disorders in bone marrow transplantation clinical evaluation with taste solutions in autologous and allogeneic bone marrow recipients, aematologica, 76(6): 519-522, 1991.

24 Ikeda K: Educational course on oral side effects of radiation therapy, Japanese Pediatric Radiation Technology, 30: 17-21, 2005.

25 Johnson ML, Farmer ER: Graft-versus-host reactions in dermatology, Journal of the American Academy of Dermatology, 38(3): 369-92, 1998. quiz 93-96. Epub 1998/03/31.

26 Hill GR, Ferrara JL: The primacy of the gastrointestinal tract as a target organ of acute graft-versus-host disease rationale for the use of cytokine shields in allogeneic bone marrow transplantation, Blood, 95(9): 2754-2759, 2000. Epub 2000/04/26.

27 Woo SB, Lee SJ, Schubert MM: Graft-vs-host disease, Critical reviews in oral biology and medicine an official publication of the American Association of Oral Biologists, 8(2): 201-216, 1997. Epub 1997/01/01.

28 Sale GE, Shulman HM, Schubert MM, Sullivan KM, Kopecky KJ, Hackman RC, et al: Oral and ophthalmic pathology of graft versus host disease in man predictive value of the lip biopsy, Human pathology, 12(11): 1022-1030, 1981. Epub 1981/11/01.

29 Lee SJ, Kim HT, Ho VT, Cutler C, Alyea EP, Soiffer RJ, et al: Quality of life associated with acute and chronic graft-versus-host disease, Bone marrow transplantation, 38(4): 305-310, 2006. Epub 2006/07/05.

30 Kadowaki K, Toyoshima T: Pathogenesis of chronic GVHD in hematopoietic stem cell transplantation, Department of Clinical Immunology and Allergy, 53(3): 337-42, 2010.

31 Shlomchik WD, Couzens MS, Tang CB, McNiff J, Robert ME, Liu J, et al: Prevention of graft versus host disease by inactivation of host antigen-presenting cells, Science, 285(5426): 412-415, 1999. Epub 1999/07/20.

32 Ferrara JL, Reddy P: Pathophysiology of graft-versus-host disease, Seminars in hematology, 43(1):

3-10, 2006. Epub 2006/01/18.

33 Schubert MM, Sullivan KM, Morton TH, Izutsu KT, Peterson DE, Flournoy N, et al: Oral

manifestations of chronic graft-v-host disease, Archives of internal medicine, 144(8): 1591-1595,

1984. Epub 1984/08/01.

34 Schubert MM, Sullivan KM: Recognition incidence and management of oral graft-versus-host disease,

NCI Monogr, (9): 135-143, 1990. Epub 1990/01/01.

35 Cunningham BA, Lenssen P, Aker SN, Gittere KM, Cheney CL, Hutchison MM: Nutritional

considerations during marrow transplantation, The Nursing clinics of North America, 18(3): 585-596,

1983. Epub 1983/09/01.

36 Fox PC: Salivary enhancement therapies, Caries research, 38(3): 241-246, 2004. Epub 2004/05/22.

37 Forman SJ: Hematopoietic cell transplantation, Second edition ed, Blackwell scientific publications,

Boston, 515-536, 1999.

38 Morishima Y, Sasazuki T, Inoko H, Juji T, Akaza T, Yamamoto K, et al: The clinical significance of

human leukocyte antigen (HLA) allele compatibility in patients receiving a marrow transplant from

serologically HLA-A HLA-B and HLA-DR matched unrelated donors, Blood, 99(11): 4200-4206,

2002. Epub 2002/05/16.

39 Nin T, Sakagami M: Taste disorder and saliva secretion disorder, ENTONI, 117: 25-30, 2010.

40 Kamikawa Y, Nagayama T, Kanekawa A, Hara K: Update on oral infections, Oral candidiasis, Dental

care, 24: 24-30, 2010.

41 Demarosi F, Lodi G, Carrassi A, Soligo D, Sardella A: Oral malignancies following HSCT graft versus

host disease and other risk factors, Oral oncology, 41(9): 865-877, 2005. Epub 2005/08/09.

42 Demarosi F, Soligo D, Lodi G, Moneghini L, Sardella A, Carrassi A: Squamous cell carcinoma of

the oral cavity associated with graft versus host disease: report of a case and review of the literature,

Oral surgery oral medicine oral pathology oral radiology and endodontics, 100(1): 63-69. 2005. Epub

2005/06/15.

43 Gallagher G, Forrest DL: Second solid cancers after allogeneic hematopoietic stem cell transplantation,

Cancer, 109(1): 84-92, 2007. Epub 2006/11/30.

Chapter 4 Oral Adverse Events

44 Curtis RE, Metayer C, Rizzo JD, Socie G, Sobocinski KA, Flowers ME, et al: Impact of chronic

GVHD therapy on the development of squamous-cell cancers after hematopoietic stem-cell

transplantation an international case-control study, Blood, 105(10): 3802-3811, 2005. Epub 2005/02/03.

Chapter **5**

Prevention of Oral Adverse Events

Chapter 5 Prevention of Oral Adverse Events

1. Preventive Strategies for Oral Adverse Events (Overview)

Oral adverse events, including oral mucositis, are influenced by various factors such as the method of hematopoietic stem cell transplantation (HSCT), the type of chemotherapy drugs used, and whether radiation therapy is administered. Unfortunately, there is currently no guaranteed method to prevent these events. However, many studies have been conducted to mitigate mucositis and oral infections, some of which provide high levels of evidence.

1) MASCC Clinical Guidelines

In 2004, the Mucositis Study Group of the Multinational Association of Supportive Care in Cancer (MASCC) and the International Society for Oral Oncology (ISOO) summarized the pathophysiology and epidemiology of mucositis[1], as well as its assessment methods, and created evidence-based clinical guidelines for mucositis management[2]. These guidelines were updated in 2007 to include additional recommendations. The guidelines for preventing oral mucositis caused by chemotherapy and radiation therapy include[3]:

1. Creation of an oral care protocol, including patient and staff education (oral hygiene guidance)

2. Use of soft toothbrushes

3. Use of patient controlled analgesia with morphine (PCA)

Additionally, for patients undergoing Hematopoietic stem cell transplantation (HSCT), which involves high-dose chemotherapy (and possibly radiation therapy), the guidelines recommend: (Table5)

1. Administration of keratinocyte growth factor (KGF-1)

2. Cryotherapy for patients receiving melphalan

1. Preventive Strategies for Oral Adverse Events (Overview)

3. Use of low-level laser therapy

Following these evidence-based guidelines has been reported to reduce oral mucositis and other adverse events[4], making preventive strategies a crucial aspect of oral care during HSCT.

Table 5 Clinical guidelines for oral care for patients with oral mucositis (2007 update)

Basic oral care and clinical practices
1 To reduce oral mucositis caused by chemotherapy and radiotherapy, we recommend creating an oral care protocol that includes education for patients and staff. In this protocol, we recommend switching to a toothbrush with softer bristles than regular ones. Appropriate clinical practice should also include the use of valid tools for the constant assessment of oral pain and condition. It is necessary that dental intervention continues throughout the treatment and follow-up period. 2 Patient-controlled analgesia (PCA) using morphine is recommended as a treatment option for oral mucositis pain in patients undergoing hematopoietic cell transplantation. It is also fundamental to enable patients to evaluate and report oral pain themselves.
High-dose chemotherapy with or without total body irradiation plus HSCT : Prevention
3 For patients with hematological malignancies undergoing high-dose chemotherapy and whole-body irradiation during autologous transplantation, keratinocyte growth factor-1 (Palifermin) was administered at 60μg/kg/day for 3 days before pretreatment and for 3 days after transplantation to prevent oral mucositis. 4 We recommend cryotherapy for oral mucosal prophylaxis in patients receiving large doses of melphalan. 5 We do not recommend using Pentoxifylline (a drug that improves cerebral circulation and metabolism) to prevent oral mucositis in patients undergoing HSTC. 6 We do not recommend the use of GM-CSF mouthwash to prevent oral mucositis in patients undergoing HSTC. 7 We recommend the use of low-power lasers to reduce oral mucositis and associated pain in patients receiving high-dose chemotherapy or chemotherapy with radiation prior to HSTC. However, low-power lasers are expensive and require special training, so they are limited to facilities that can do this. This is because treatment results vary depending on the skill of the surgeon, making it difficult to summarize the results of clinical trials. However, I hope that evidence supporting this will continue to accumulate.

Refer Keefe D et al: Updated clinical practice guidelines for the prevention andtreatment of mucositis, Cancer, 109(5):820~831, 2007

Chapter 5 Prevention of Oral Adverse Events

2) Guidelines in Japan

The MASCC guidelines are based on evidence from international studies and may not be directly applicable in Japan. In particular, the approval status of medications used for prevention, such as keratinocyte growth factor (Palifermin) or the antioxidant Amifostine, differs in Japan, where these drugs have not been approved. Therefore, we believe that while referencing international guidelines, we need to develop a set of guidelines tailored to Japan's circumstances.

When creating these guidelines, it is essential to present "recommended" practices based on evidence from both domestic and international literature. However, since this alone may provide limited guidance for healthcare providers and patients involved in HSCT, we will also introduce studies with valuable insights, even if their evidence is not fully established, as "background" information. Guidelines should be regularly updated based on new research[5], and it is important to share them widely with all stakeholders and ensure their application in clinical settings.

2. Efficacy of Oral Care as Prevention of Oral Adverse Events

1) Recommended Practice

For HSCT patients, oral care including brushing and mouth rinsing is effective in preventing oral mucositis and may reduce the occurrence of secondary bacteremia and sepsis.

2) Evidence (Background)

Numerous reports have shown that dental visits before chemotherapy and radiation therapy, along with brushing and mouth rinsing to control plaque, are effective as preventive measures for oral mucositis. In the 1980s, Sonis et al.[6] reported that 40% of non-head and neck cancer patients experienced oral discomfort, but proactive dental intervention could reduce these issues. The 1989 NIH consensus conference emphasized that all cancer patients should receive dental care before undergoing chemotherapy or radiation, and that dentists, dental hygienists, and caregivers should learn about oral adverse events related to cancer treatment[7].

(1) Oral Care for Mucositis Prevention

Studies have explored whether oral care is effective in preventing mucositis in cancer patients, including those with leukemia. Carl[8] reported that oral care and dental treatment were effective for alleviating oral discomfort, and Levy-Polack[9] showed that in children with acute lymphoblastic leukemia (ALL), continuous oral care with brushing and mouth rinses reduced the severity of mucositis. Cheng et al.[10,11] reported that oral care education in pediatric patients with blood cancers was challenging, but adhering to detailed oral care instructions during chemotherapy reduced mucositis symptoms and pain.

McGuire et al.[12] confirmed the MASCC guidelines for mucositis prevention, emphasizing the importance of oral hygiene education, soft toothbrushes, PCA for pain management, and pre-treatment dental care. Djuric[13] reported that pre-treatment dental care, plaque control, and tartar removal were effective in reducing mucositis scores. Ohbayashi et al.[14] found that cryotherapy with ice chips was insufficient as a preventive measure, but oral healthcare was effective.

However, while oral care can reduce mucositis, completely preventing it remains challenging. Santos[15] reported that although oral care could not reduce the frequency of mucositis, it could shorten the duration of patient suffering.

(2) Prevention of Bacteremia and Sepsis

Greenberg et al.[16,17] found that bacteremia and sepsis in leukemia treatment could be linked to oral infections, and that dental care before chemotherapy could reduce these risks. Borrowski[18] found that while aggressive oral cleaning and dental care reduced mucositis, it

Chapter 5 Prevention of Oral Adverse Events

did not prevent sepsis.

(3) Effectiveness of Oral Care

Although it is difficult to prevent oral mucositis entirely, based on previous reports, we recommend early, appropriate, and continuous oral care to reduce the severity of adverse events, alleviate patient discomfort, shorten their duration, and possibly reduce hospitalization time.

3. Flow of Prevention Strategies for Oral Adverse Events

1) Recommended Practices

Oral care for preventing oral adverse events should follow a sequence across the stages of HSCT treatment as follows:

(1) Pre-treatment Prevention

· Oral assessment and examination

· Education on the importance of oral care

· Instruction on oral hygiene and tartar removal

· Prioritization of dental treatments to eliminate infection sources

(2) Pre-conditioning to Engraftment

· Continuation of oral hygiene

· Ongoing assessments

· Management of adverse events (mucosal protection, pain relief, moisturizing, infection prevention)

(3) Post-engraftment GvHD Prevention

· Continued oral care

48

・Regular dental check-ups

・Focus on infection prevention

・Dietary advice

The most critical strategy is preparing the oral environment before starting pre-conditioning to minimize the damage caused by chemotherapy and radiation[19].

2) Evidence (Background)

Patients diagnosed with blood diseases such as leukemia or lymphoma may undergo high-dose chemotherapy and radiation before receiving HSCT, leading to significant immune suppression. Oral adverse events, especially mucositis, are most prominent during this period, so it is essential to complete most preventive measures before pre-conditioning begins.

Prevention of infections, removal of irritants that exacerbate mucosal damage, and pain relief are the three major pillars of oral care. Infection prevention and irritant removal must be initiated early and continued throughout the treatment.

Specific preventive strategies include:

① Creation of protocols to monitor and assess patient conditions and share information across teams

② Improving patient motivation for oral care and providing oral hygiene guidance

③ Dental treatments before pre-conditioning

④ Cryotherapy

⑤ Drug-based preventive measures

⑥ Dietary guidance

⑦ Others (Use of protective devices, mouthguards, fluoride, and prevention of mouth opening issues)

Chapter 5 Prevention of Oral Adverse Events

4. Oral Hygiene Instruction

1) Plaque Control

(1) Recommended Points

For plaque control, the following points are recommended:

① Pre-transplant brushing education: Before undergoing chemotherapy or radiation therapy, it is essential for dentists and dental hygienists to provide brushing instruction, ensuring that patients and caregivers receive thorough education.

② Brushing methods: There is limited evidence on the most recommended brushing methods, but continuous brushing throughout the treatment period is considered important in preventing oral mucositis.

③ When brushing is difficult due to oral mucositis: When oral mucositis is present, and brushing with a regular toothbrush is difficult, the use of soft brushes, super-soft brushes, or sponge brushes should be recommended.

④ Dry mouth management: If dry mouth is present, mouth rinses or moisturizers should be used alongside brushing.

(2) Evidence (Background)

Many facilities have reported efforts for oral care in patients undergoing HSCT, but evidence-based methods have not yet been established. Schubert et al.[20] emphasize the importance of initiating oral care before transplant and providing oral hygiene instructions throughout the transplant period to address the various oral conditions at each stage.

① Brushing Methods

The National Cancer Institute (NCI) recommends brushing with a soft nylon toothbrush (2-3 rows) using the Bass method, aimed at plaque removal from the gingival sulcus, and performing it 2-3 times a day[21]. If the patient can use it safely without causing injury, an

50

electric toothbrush or ultrasonic toothbrush may also be used. Additionally, rinsing with water or saline 3-4 times while brushing may enhance the plaque removal effect. Alcohol-based mouthwashes should be avoided.

When selecting toothpaste, it is advisable to choose one with minimal flavoring, as some may irritate oral soft tissues. Brushing should be followed by rinsing the toothbrush with hot water every 15-30 seconds to soften the bristles and reduce the risk of trauma. After use, the toothbrush should be air-dried.

For interdental cleaning, if the patient can safely use dental floss without injuring the gum tissue, it may continue throughout the chemotherapy period. Flossing can help remove bacterial plaque from interdental spaces and improve gum health. Both brushing and interdental cleaning should be performed under the supervision of specialized staff.

Regarding the use of sponge brushes, Bavier[22] and Baddour et al.[23] suggest that when oral mucositis makes regular brushing difficult, sponge brushes or ultra-soft brushes soaked in chlorhexidine can be used for cleaning. However, NCI[21] reports that sponge brushes are ineffective for cleaning teeth and should not replace regular soft-bristled toothbrushes, particularly since rough sponge surfaces may irritate and damage the mucosal surfaces opposite the teeth.

Other oral care recommendations include avoiding the use of toothpicks or water-pick devices during immunosuppressive periods, as stated by Schulbert et al.[20] and Little et al.[24].

② Moisturization Methods

For dry mouth, in addition to moisturizers, artificial saliva may be considered. Tsukuda et al.[25] compared spray-type artificial saliva and a glycerol-based moisturizer and found that the moisturizer had better usability and longer-lasting hydration. Other studies have also reported the effectiveness of glycerol-based moisturizers[26-30]. According to Yamano et al.[30], applying moisturizers after brushing or rinsing helps retain moisture in the mouth,

Chapter 5 Prevention of Oral Adverse Events

improving the oral environment and alleviating patients' symptoms.

Regarding actual use, Mogi et al.[31] reported using mouth rinses and gels prophylactically from the onset of mucosal swelling due to chemotherapy, before the formation of mucosal lesions on the tongue and buccal mucosa.

As noted earlier, while effective oral care to prevent the various adverse events in the oral cavity has not been fully established, we recommend providing appropriate oral hygiene instructions early on, continuing throughout the treatment period, as this may reduce the severity of adverse events, alleviate patient discomfort, shorten the duration of symptom onset, and possibly shorten hospitalization.

2) Mouth Rinsing

(1) Recommended Points

Although there is no established evidence regarding the effectiveness of various mouthwashes, it is believed that mouth rinsing throughout the treatment period can be effective for moisturizing the mouth and for antibacterial and disinfectant effects.

(2) Evidence (Background)

① Chlorhexidine

Much of the research on mouthwashes overseas has focused on chlorhexidine. The effectiveness of chlorhexidine mouthwashes has been discussed in many studies over the years. Addy et al.[32] measured bacterial counts in saliva after using various concentrations of chlorhexidine mouthwash, showing that the formulation affected its antimicrobial persistence. Ferretti et al.[33,34] reported that using 0.12% chlorhexidine gluconate mouthwash could reduce mucosal damage in patients undergoing intensive chemotherapy. Rutkauskas et al.[35] demonstrated the effectiveness of chlorhexidine in bone marrow transplant patients, while Costa et al.[36] found it beneficial for pediatric patients with acute lymphoblastic leukemia.

However, there are also reports suggesting that chlorhexidine mouthwashes may not significantly prevent mucositis compared to control groups[37], and other studies have concluded that chlorhexidine is ineffective for mucositis prevention[38-41]. As such, there is no conclusive evidence on the efficacy of chlorhexidine in preventing oral mucositis, and the MASCC guidelines currently exclude it from recommended practices.

② Other Mouthwashes

In Japan, facilities often recommend mouthwashes with sodium azulene sulfonate, saline, or iodine gargles over chlorhexidine. Povidone-iodine has strong antibacterial properties[42-44] and can reduce bacterial counts, but it does not have plaque-removal effects. It tends to lose its antibacterial effect over time, and there are mixed reports regarding its duration of effect. Additionally, because it contains alcohol, it can irritate mucosal surfaces, making it unsuitable for use during mucositis[45,46]. Furthermore, it is contraindicated in patients with thyroid disorders or iodine sensitivity.

As a result, many facilities use sodium azulene sulfonate. While it does not have antibacterial properties, it promotes wound healing and has anti-inflammatory effects[47,48]. It is often used in gargles or as a mouthwash combined with baking soda (2%) to treat oral dryness and mucositis. Sodium azulene sulfonate is favored because it is easy to use even when the patient experiences nausea or mucositis[49,50].

If nausea is severe or mucositis prevents the use of azulene mouthwash, saline is used instead[46]. Although initially salty, saline is less irritating and painless to rinse with.

Recently, there has been increasing research into more effective mouthwash methods using green tea or lemon water, and many facilities have developed original mouthwash solutions that are easier for patients to use without causing discomfort.

If adverse events such as mucositis occur and pain management is needed,

Chapter 5 Prevention of Oral Adverse Events

mouthwashes with azulene or saline can be combined with anesthetics like xylocaine to help alleviate pain, as discussed in another section.

Although many studies have explored the efficacy of mouthwashes, conclusive evidence is still lacking. However, rather than focusing on the selection of mouthwashes, it is crucial to ensure that mouth rinsing is performed at least 5-8 times a day to maintain oral hydration and cleansing, which is a guideline recommendation.

5. Dental Treatment to Be Performed Before Transplantation

1) Recommended Items

Dental foci can be a potential source of systemic infection, so they should be removed or improved before starting chemotherapy.

(1) Guidelines for the Treatment of Caries and Pulpitis

For mild to moderate caries, if time permits, restorative procedures should be carried out; if there is not enough time, observation should be performed. However, to prevent irritation caused by sharp edges of teeth resulting from caries, at least temporary fillings or provisional sealing should be done. In cases of severe caries associated with pulpitis, the tooth should either be extracted or, if time allows, pulp therapy should be performed to preserve the tooth as much as possible.

(2) Guidelines for the Treatment of Apical Periodontitis

If no symptoms are present and the radiolucency at the apex is small, observation is acceptable. If the radiolucency exceeds 5mm, root canal therapy should be performed if time allows; otherwise, extraction is the basic option. If symptoms are present, root canal treatment should be performed if sufficient time is available, but extraction is often the first choice.

(3) Guidelines for the Treatment of Marginal Periodontitis

Teeth showing acute symptoms should be extracted before transplantation. Even if there are no symptoms, if the periodontal pockets are deep and significant mobility is present, extraction is recommended. In other cases, efforts should be made to improve the condition through tartar removal and oral hygiene education.

(4) Guidelines for the Extraction of Wisdom Teeth

For asymptomatic wisdom teeth, observation without treatment is recommended. If symptoms are present, extraction should only be performed if there is sufficient healing time after the procedure.

2) Evidence (Background)

As mentioned earlier, immune suppression associated with transplantation or radiation therapy can lead to a secondary state of immunosuppression, making the body more susceptible to infections, sometimes even leading to sepsis and threatening life. Since the oral cavity is a major route for pathogens to enter the body, maintaining oral hygiene and removing potential oral infection sources, i.e., performing dental treatment before transplantation, are crucial[6,51-53]. According to NIH consensus, "Dental foci can be a potential source of systemic infection, and should be removed or improved before starting chemotherapy"[54]. Therefore, to prevent severe systemic infections, it is necessary to identify potential infection sources through pre-transplant screening and provide appropriate treatment[55].

At the same time, the reality is that the period available for dental treatment before transplantation is limited[56]. Some studies indicate that dental treatment does not significantly affect the prognosis of cancer treatment[57], and others report no significant difference in the incidence of oral infections during or after HSCT. Thus, only minimal treatment targeting

Chapter 5 Prevention of Oral Adverse Events

potential infection sources should be performed. Additionally, to minimize the reduction in quality of life (QOL) and ensure proper healing time after extraction, unnecessary extractions of teeth that can be preserved should be avoided. Therefore, we recommend conducting adequate dental screenings, creating management protocols considering the timing of transplantation[59], and prioritizing the removal of infection sources before transplantation, while performing conservative dental treatments whenever possible.

Potential sources of infection in the oral cavity include caries, the pulpitis that follows, apical periodontitis, periodontitis (marginal periodontitis), and semi-impacted wisdom teeth.

(1) Treatment of Caries and Pulpitis

The guidelines for caries from Peterson et al.[52], Yamagata et al.,[59] and the American Academy of Pediatric Dentistry[60] are summarized as follows:

- For mild to moderate caries (C1-C2) without symptoms, either observation with temporary restoration (provisional sealing) or restorative treatment if time allows should be performed. Sharp edges of teeth caused by caries must be removed to prevent irritation to the mucosa.

- For advanced caries leading to pulpitis (C3), if sufficient time is available, root canal therapy should be performed; if time is limited, extraction may be considered.

- For teeth with advanced decay (C4), extraction is usually performed, but if extraction cannot be done due to time or blood test results, at least removal of infected dental material and temporary root surface restoration to avoid irritation is necessary.

- Research has been conducted on the use of fluoride and chlorhexidine for the prevention or progression control of early caries, but the evidence is insufficient to recommend them.

(2) Treatment of Apical Periodontitis

It was previously believed that teeth with apical lesions should be proactively extracted before transplantation to prevent post-transplant infections, but it is now recognized that root canal therapy can often preserve the tooth, especially under time constraints[61]. Furthermore, considering the risks of pre-transplant extractions, treatment should focus on preserving the tooth as much as possible. Whether or not there are symptoms, or whether the X-ray shows a radiolucent lesion at the apex, greatly influences the treatment approach. There are reports stating that if no symptoms are observed at all, the occurrence of infectious complications during HSCT treatment is not affected even without treatment[62], and there are also reports indicating that no cases of acute transformation of periapical lesions with less than 2mm radiolucency have been observed during HSCT treatment[59], so if the radiolucency is 5mm or less, active root canal treatment may not be necessary. If it exceeds 5mm, root canal therapy should be performed if time allows, or extraction may be necessary. In the presence of acute symptoms such as swelling, pain, or pus, extraction is often required. If there is sufficient time before transplantation, efforts should be made to preserve the tooth with root canal therapy, but extraction should be considered if the prognosis is poor.

(3) Treatment of Marginal Periodontitis

Marginal periodontitis (periodontal disease) is the most common infection in adult oral cavities and is one of the most likely infectious complications during HSCT therapy[63]. However, since it often shows a chronic course, determining its significance as an infection source can be difficult. If there are signs of periodontal pockets, tooth mobility, or bleeding, extraction is recommended if the risk of infection is high during periods of immune suppression. Generally, if acute symptoms such as spontaneous pain, biting pain, gum swelling, or pus/bleeding from periodontal pockets are present, extraction should be performed before transplantation.

Even in the absence of symptoms, there are mixed reports regarding whether extraction should be proactively recommended[64-67]. In this guideline, it is recommended to extract

Chapter 5 Prevention of Oral Adverse Events

teeth with significant periodontal pocket depth or mobility, even if there are no symptoms. Otherwise, efforts should be made to improve the condition through tartar removal and oral hygiene education, with extraction considered if no improvement is seen.

(4) Extraction of Wisdom Teeth

The approach to the extraction of semi-impacted or fully impacted wisdom teeth varies, with some recommending proactive extraction[64,65] and others advocating for caution[66,67]. We recommend observation without treatment for asymptomatic wisdom teeth, and extraction should only be performed if there is enough healing time post-extraction.

(5) Pediatric Patients and Treatment of Deciduous Teeth

Generally, adult guidelines can be applied to pediatric patients, but because symptoms may become acute more easily in children, extra caution should be taken regarding infection prevention. If there is sufficient time before transplantation, it may be better to choose extraction for teeth with even a small concern about prognosis.

For patients wearing orthodontic appliances, it is better to remove them to prevent the worsening of any potential infections. Removable appliances may be continued if possible.

6. Cryotherapy

1) Recommended Items

In cases where high doses of 5-FU (fluorouracil) or melphalan are administered, cryotherapy has been reported to reduce the incidence and severity of oral mucositis. However, due to insufficient evidence, it is not currently recommended.

2) Evidence (Background)

Cryotherapy involves cooling the oral cavity during chemotherapy to constrict local blood vessels, reducing the migration of anticancer agents to the oral mucosa and alleviating oxidative stress from free radicals, thus preventing oral mucositis[68-72]. Cryotherapy is inexpensive and well-tolerated. The method involves holding ice chips, ice balls, or cold water in the mouth for 5 minutes before chemotherapy, during chemotherapy, and for 15-30 minutes after chemotherapy[69]. Studies by Mahood et al.[68] and Lilleby et al.[70] showed a significant reduction in the incidence of oral mucositis with cryotherapy in patients receiving high doses of 5-FU and melphalan, respectively. However, the mechanism needs further investigation. Mori et al.[73] have made similar reports in cases of high-dose cytarabine administration, but they note that the mechanism of its occurrence needs to be examined in the future. On the other hand, Gori et al.[74] reported that cryotherapy was not effective in preventing oral mucositis in patients receiving methotrexate post-bone marrow transplantation. The current evidence on cryotherapy remains insufficient. According to the MASCC guidelines, cryotherapy is recommended only for bolus administration of 5-FU, edatrexate, or high-dose melphalan.

Chapter 5 Prevention of Oral Adverse Events

7. Systemic Adverse Events such as Bacteremia and Sepsis

1) Recommended Items

The oral cavity contains numerous resident bacteria, periodontal disease-related bacteria, and endodontic pathogens, so it is important to prevent infections from occurring at mucositis sites. While there is no definitive consensus, removing oral infection sources and preventing or minimizing the severity of mucositis during the neutropenic phase of hematopoietic stem cell transplantation (HSCT) is important for preventing bacteremia, sepsis, and other systemic adverse events. Therefore, it is recommended to perform dental treatment to remove oral infection sources before chemotherapy and continuous oral care before and after transplantation.

2) Evidence (Background)

Reports questioning the necessity of dental treatment prior to hematopoietic stem cell transplantation (HSCT) have been made for various reasons, including the fact that cancer treatment outcomes are not affected by the presence or exacerbation of chronic dental diseases[57], and that there is no significant difference in the frequency of post-transplant infections based on whether or not dental treatment is performed[58]. On the other hand, there are reports indicating that performing oral care and removing oral infection sources before HSCT can prevent the occurrence of oral infections[59], and thus, no clear consensus has been reached on the matter.

Additionally, reports suggest that the implementation of oral management during HSCT contributes to a reduction in the incidence of oral mucositis and pneumonia post-transplantation[75, 76]. It has also been reported that patients with periodontal disease tend to have higher CRP levels, but these levels significantly decrease following periodontal treatment[77].

As mentioned earlier, approximately 80% of hematopoietic stem cell transplant patients develop oral mucositis, which is known to cause not only bacteremia and sepsis but also issues such as changes in treatment plans and increased medical costs[78]. For various infection prevention measures in stem cell transplantation, fluoroquinolone antibiotics, antifungals, and antivirals are generally administered. During the neutropenic phase associated with HSCT, endogenous infections in the gastrointestinal tract, which suffers mucosal damage due to pre-transplant conditioning, become problematic, and sepsis caused by Gram-negative bacteria, particularly Pseudomonas aeruginosa, is reported to be fatal[79]. The Japanese Society for Hematopoietic Stem Cell Transplantation also recommends careful determination of drug use, considering the risk of resistant bacteria from prophylactic administration, with attention to individual facilities and patients[80]. However, there are no reports linking oral diseases to bacteremia or sepsis, and it is believed that preventing the onset of conditions like oral mucositis and their severe progression during the neutropenic phase of transplantation will subsequently prevent secondary systemic adverse events.

(Junpei Sugisaki, Department of Dentistry, Toranomon Hospital

Akiko Abe, Department of Preventive Dentistry, Faculty of Dentistry, Iwate Medical University

Takae Abe, Department of Geriatric Dentistry, Hokkaido University Hospital)

References

1 Sonis ST, Elting LS, Keefe D, et al: Perspectives on cancer therapy-induced mucosal injury pathogenesis measurement epidemiology and consequences for patients, Cancer, 100(9 suppl): 1995-2025, 2004.

2 Rubenstein EB, Peterson DE, Schubert M, et al: Clinical practice guidelines for the prevention and treatment of cancer therapy-induced oral and gastrointestinal mucositis, Cancer, 100(9 suppl): 2026-2046, 2004.

3 Keefe D, Schubert M, Elting LS, et al: Updated clinical practice guidelines for the prevention and treatment of mucositis, Cancer, 109(5): 820-831, 2007.

4 Brennan MT, Bültzingslöwen I, Schubert MM, Keefe D: Alimentary mucositis: putting the guidelines into practice, Support Care Cancer, 14: 573-579, 2006.

5 Keefe D: Mucositis guidelines: what have they achieved, and where to from here?, Support Care Cancer, 14: 489-491, 2006.

6 Sonis S, Kunz A: Impact of improved dental services on the frequency of oral complications of cancer therapy for patients with non-head-and-neck malignancies, Oral Surg Oral Med Oral Pathol, 65(1): 19-22, 1988.

7 National Institutes of Health Consensus development conference statement oral complications of cancer therapies: diagnosis, prevention, and treatment, National Institutes of Health, Bethesda Md, 1989.

8 Carl W: Oral complications of local and systemic cancer treatment, Curr Opin Oncol, 7(4): 320-324, 1995.

9 Levy-Polack MP, Sebelli P, Polack NL: Incidence of oral complications and application of a preventive protocol in children with acute leukemia, Spec Care Dentist, 18(5): 189-193, 1998.

10 Cheng KK, Molassiotis A, Chang AM, Wai WC, Cheung SS: Evaluation of an oral care protocol intervention in the prevention of chemotherapy-induced oral mucositis in pediatric cancer patients, Eur J Cancer, 37(16): 2056-2063, 2001.

11 Cheng KK, Molassiotis A, Chang AM: An oral care protocol intervention to prevent chemotherapy-

induced oral mucositis in paediatric cancer patients: a pilot study, Eur J Oncol Nurs, 6(2): 66-73, 2002.

12　McGuire DB, Correa ME, Johnson J, Wienandts P: The role of basic oral care and good clinical practice principles in the management of oral mucositis, Support Care Cancer, 14(6): 541-547, 2006.

13　Djuric M, Kolarov V, Bellic A, Jankovic L: Mucositis prevention by improved dental care in acute leukemia patients, Support Care Cancer, 14(2): 137-146, 2006.

14　Ohbayashi Y, Imataki O, Ohnishi H, et al: Multivariate analysis of factors influencing oral mucositis in allogeneic hematopoietic stem cell transplantation, Ann Hematol, 87: 837-845, 2008.

15　Santos PS, Coracin FL, Barros JCA, Dulley FL, Nunes FD, Magalhäes MG: Impact of oral care prior to HSCT on the severity and clinical outcomes of oral mucositis, Clin Transplant, 25(2): 325-328, 2011.

16　Greenberg MS, Cohen SG, McKitrick JC, Cassileth PA: The oral flor as a source of septicemia in patients with acute leukemia, Oral Surg Oral Med Oral Pathol, 53(1): 32-36, 1982.

17　Greenberg MS: Prechemotherapy dental treatment to prevent bacteremia, NCL Monogr, (9): 49-50, 1990.

18　Borowski B, Benhamou E, Pico JL, Laplanche A, Margainaud JP, Hayat M: Prevention of oral mucositis in patients treated with high-dose chemotherapy and bone marow transplantation: a randomised controlled trial comparing two protocols of dental care, Eur J Cancer B Oral Oncol, 30B (2): 93-97, 1994.

19　Ota Y: Oral care for patients undergoing hematopoietic stem cell transplantation, Nursing techniques, 52: 1270-1273, 2006.

20　Schubert MM, Peterson DE: Oral complications of hematopoietic cell transplantation Thomas' Hematopoietic Cell Transplantation Stem Cell Transplantation, 4th ed, Wiley-Blackwell, Oxford UK, 1589-1607, 2009.

21　National Cancer Institute: Oral Complications of Chemotherapy and Head/Neck Radiation (PDQ®), National Cancer Institute, Bethesda, 2011.

22　Bavier AR: Nursing management of acute oral complications of cancer, NCI Monogr, 9: 123-128, 1990.

23　Baddour LM, Bettman MA, Bolger AF, et al: Nonvalvular cardiovascular device-related infection,

Chapter 5 Prevention of Oral Adverse Events

Circ, 108(16): 2015-2031, 2003.

24 Little JW, Falace DA, Miller CS, Rhodus Nl: Dental Manegement of the medically Compromised Patient, 7th ed, Mo Mosby, St Louis, 433-461, 2008.

25 Tsunoda H, Niisato C, Wakabayashi R, et al: Effects of Oral Balance BioTeen Gel on patients with Sjögren's syndrome, Dental Diamond, 10: 158-161, 2001.

26 Morita Y, et al: Usefulness of oral balance for dry mouth in preoperative patients, Anesthesia, 53: 772-776, 2004.

27 Regelink G, et al: Efficacy of a synthetic polymer saliva substitute in reducing oral complaints of patients suffering from irradiation-induced xerostomia, Quintessence Int, 29: 383-388, 1998.

28 Yamamoto K, et al: Effect of moisturizing gel on patients with dry mouth, Journal of Oral Mucosa, 11: 1-7, 2005.

29 Ishimaru T: Radiation therapy and xerostomia, ENTONI, 65: 37-41, 2006.

30 Yamano T, et al: The usefulness of oral balance for dry mouth during radiotherapy for head and neck cancer, 54(1): 37-40, 2008.

31 Mogi N, Ikegami Y, Narita K, et al: Effect of oral care on hematopoietic cell transplant patients on length of hospital stay, Journal of the Japanese Oral Care Society, 1(1): 14-20, 2007.

32 Addy M, Jenkins S, Newcombe R: The effect of some chlorhexidine-containing mouthrinses on salivary bacterial counts, J Clin Periodontol, 18: 90-93, 1991.

33 Ferretti GA, Ash RC, Brown AT, Largent BM, Kaplan A, Lillich TT: Chlorhexidine for prophylaxis against oral infections and associated complications in patients receiving bone marrow transplants, J Am Dent Assoc, 114: 461-467, 1987.

34 Ferretti GA, Raybould TP, Brown AT, Macdonald JS, Greenwood M, Maruyama Y, Gcil J, Lillich TT, Ash RC: Chlorhexidine prophylaxis for chemotherapy and radiotherapy-induced stomatitis: a randomized double-blind trial, Oral Surg Oral Med Oral Pathol, 69: 331-338, 1990.

35 Rutkauskas JS, Davis JW: Effects of chlorhexidine during immunosuppressive chemotherapy. A preliminary report, Oral Surg Oral Med Oral Pathol, 76: 441-448, 1993.

36 Costa EM, Fernandes MZ, Quindere LB, de Souza LB, Pinto LP: Evaluation of an oral preventive protocol in children with acute lymphoblastic leukemia, Pesqui Odontol Bras, 17: 147-150, 2003.

37 Lanzos I, Herrera D, Santos S, O'Connor A, Pena C, Lanzos E, Sanz M: Mucositis in irradiated cancer patients: Effects of an antiseptic mouthrinse, Med Oral Pathol Oral Cir Bucal, 15: e732-738, 2010.

38 Wahlin YB: Effects of chlorhexidine mouthrinse on oral health in patients with acute leukemia, Oral Surg Oral Med Oral Pathol, 68: 279-287, 1989.

39 Foote RL, Loprinzi CL, Frank AR, O'Fallon JR, Gulavita S, Tewfik HH, Ryan MA, Earle JM, Novotny P: Randomized trial of a chlorhexidine mouthwash for alleviation of radiation-induced mucositis, J Clin Oncol, 12: 2630-2633, 1994.

40 Dodd MJ, Larson PJ, Dibble SL, Miaskowski C, Greenspan D, MacPhail L, Hauck WW, Paul SM, Ignoffo R, Shiba G: Randomized clinical trial of chlorhexidine versus placebo for prevention of oral mucositis in patients receiving chemotherapy, Oncol Nurs Forum, 23: 921-927, 1996.

41 Antunes H, Ferreira E, Faria L, Schirmer M, Rodrigues P, Small I, Colares M, Bouzas L, Ferreira C: Streptococcal bacteremia in patients submitted to hematopoietic stem cell transplantation: The role of tooth brushing and use of chlorhexidine, Med Oral Pathol Oral Cir Bucal, 15: e303-309, 2010.

42 Kamoi K, Miyata H, Ogi S, Shimizu T, Koide K, Nakajima S, Kojima T, Nishizawa S, Higashitsutsumi M, Sakamoto M, Tsuchiya T, Hatae S: In vitro treatment of oral pathogenic bacteria sterilizing effect of povidone-iodine solution, Journal of Periodontal Research, 32: 660-666, 1988.

43 Ogawa T, Konobe H, Kamoi K, Ota Y, Shimizu M, Yamada M: Effects of povidone-iodine-containing gargle (Isodyne Gurgle®) on subperiodontal bacterial flora and clinical symptoms, Journal of Periodontal Research, 38: 354-358, 1996.

44 Sasaoka K, Mogi K, Jinno K, Negishi A: Study on the effects of various oral care treatments - using oral resident bacteria as an indicator - 3rd report Effect of brushing, Kitakanto Med J, 58: 147-151, 2008.

45 Nishihira M: Oral care for hematopoietic stem cell transplant patients - How to prevent oral infections. Nursing techniques, 48: 1252-1257, 2002.

46 Yamada M: Oral care of hematopoietic stem cell transplant patients, Cancer nursing, 9: 408-414, 2004.

47 Yamazaki H et al: Pharmacology of guaiazulene, especially anti-inflammatory effect and histamine release effect, Japanese Pharmacology Journal, 53: 362-377, 1958.

Chapter 5 Prevention of Oral Adverse Events

48 Shibata Y, et al: Mechanism of anti-inflammatory action of sodium azulene sulfonate, Pharmacology and clinical, 14: 1303-1311, 1986.

49 Ota Y, Nishimura T, Zenta S: Methods for alleviating symptoms of oral mucositis using radiation therapy and chemotherapy, Nursing techniques, 52: 1264-1267, 2006.

50 Ikegami Y: Prevention of oral mucosal disorders after hematopoietic stem cell transplantation, Internal medicine, 104: 267-272, 2009.

51 Overholser CD: Periodontal infection in patients with acute non-lymphocytic leukemia. prevalence of acute exacerbations, Arch Intern Med, 142: 551-554, 1982.

52 Peterson DE: Pretreatment strategies for infection prevention in chemotherapy patients, NCL Monogr, 9: 61-71, 1990.

53 Barker GJ: Currentpractices in the oral management of the patient undergoing chemotherapy or bone marrow transplantation, Support Care Cancer, 7: 17-20, 1999.

54 Consensus statement: oral complications of cancer therapies. National Institutes of Health Consensus Development panel, NCI Monogr, 9: 3-8, 1990.

55 Bergmann O: Oral infections and septicemia in immunocompromised patients with hematologic malignancies, J Clin Microbiol, 26: 2105-2109, 1988.

56 Elad S, Garfunkel AA, Or R, Michaeli E, Shapira MY, Galili D: Time limitations and the challenge of providing infection-preventing dental care to hematopoietic stem-cell transplantation patients, Support Care Cancer, 11: 674-677, 2003.

57 Toljanic JA, Bedard JF, Larson RA, Fox JP: A prospective pilot study to evaluate a new dental assessment and treatment paradigm for patients scheduled to undergo intensive chemotherapy for cancer, Cancer, 85: 1843-1848, 1999,

58 Melkos AB, Massenkeil G, Arnold R, Reichart PA: Dental treatment prior to stem cell transplantation and its influence on the posttransplantation outcome, Clin Oral Invest, 7: 113-115, 2003.

59 Yamagata K, Onizawa K, Yanagawa T, Hasegawa Y, Kojima H, Nagasawa T, Yoshida H: A prospective study to evaluate a new dental management protocol before hematopoietic stem cell transplantation, Bone Marrow Transplantation, 38: 237-242, 2006.

60　American Academy of Pediatric Dentistry: Clinical guideline on dental management of pediatric patients receiving chemotherapy, hematopoietic cell transplantation, and/or radiation, Pediatr Dent, 26(7 Suppl): 144-149, 2004.

61　Komatsu H, Kobayashi Y, Kawakami S, Tanaka T, Noda M, Matsuda Y, Sasakawa W: Infected root canal treatment for organ transplant patients, The Japanese Journal of Conservative Dentistry, 46 (6): 845-852, 2003.

62　Peters E, Monopoli M, Woo SB, Sonis S: Assessment of the need for treatment of postendodontic asymptomatic periapical radiolucencies in bone marrow transplant recipients, Oral Surg Oral Med Oral Pathol, 76: 45-48, 1993.

63　Akintoye SO, Brennan MT, Graber CJ, Mckinney BE, Rams TE, Barret AJ, et al: A retrospective investigation of advanced periodontal disease as a risk for septicemia in hematopoietic sterm cell and bone marrow transplant recipients, Oral Surg Oral Med Oral Pathol Oral Radiol Endod, 94: 581-588, 2002.

64　Maxymiw WG, Wood RE: The role of dentistry in patients undergoing bone marrow transplantation, Br Dent J, 167: 229-233, 1989.

65　Carl W: Bone marrow transplants and oral complications, Quintessence Int, 10: 1001-1009, 1984.

66　Mercier P, Precious D: Risks and benefits of removal of impacted third molars, Int J Oral Maxillofac surg, 21: 17-27, 1992.

67　Tai CCE, Precious DS, Wood RE: Prophylactic extraction of third molars in cancer patients, Oral Surg Oral Med Oral Pathol, 78: 151-155, 1994.

68　Mahood DJ, Dose AM, Loprinzi CL, et al: Inhibition of fluorouracil-induced stomatitis by oral cryotherapy, J. Clin Oncol, 9: 449-452, 1991.

69　Aisa Y, Mori T, Kudo M, Yashima T, Kondo S, Yokoyama A, et al: Oral cryotherapy for the prevention of high-dose melphalan-induced stomatitis in sllogeneic hematopoietic stem cell transplantation, Support Care Cancer, 13: 266-269, 2005.

70　Lilleby,K, Garcia P, Gooley T, McDonnell P, Taber R, Holmberg L, et al: A prospective, randomized study of cryotherapy during administration of high-dose melphalan to decrease the severity and duration of oral mucositis in patients with multiple myeloma undergoing autologous peripheral blood

Chapter 5 Prevention of Oral Adverse Events

stem cell transplantation, Bone Marrow Transplantation, 37(11): 1031-1035, 2006.

71 Nikoletti S, Hyde S, Shaw T, Myers H, Kristjanson LJ: Comparison of plain ice and flavoured ice for preventing oral mucositis associated with the use of 5 fluorouracil, Clinical Nursing, 14(6): 750-753, 2005.

72 Tartaron A, Matera R, Romano G, Vigliotti ML, Renzo ND: Prevention of high-dose melphalan-induced mucositis by cryotherapy, Leukemia and Lymphoma, 46(4): 633-634, 2005.

73 Mori T, Hasegawa K, Okabe A, Tsujimura N, Kawata Y, Yashima T, et al: Efficacy of mouth rinse in preventing oral mucositis in patients receiving high-dose cytarabine for allogeneic hematopoietic stem cell transplantation, Int J Hematol, 88: 583-587, 2008.

74 Gori E, Arpinati M, Bonnifazi F, Errico A, Mega A, Alberani F, et al: Cryotherapy in the prevention of oral mucositis in patients receiving low-dose methotrezate following myeloablative allogeneic stem cell transplantation: a prospective randomized study of the Gruppo Italiano Trapianto di Midollo Osseo nurses group, Bone Marrow Transplantation, 39: 347-352 2007.

75 Kataoka N, Kuramoto W, Nagakura S, Hidaka M, Kiyokawa T, Kono F, Fujiyoshi F: Oral management of hematopoietic stem cell transplantation chemotherapy patients from a dental perspective, Journal of Dental Health, 55: 461, 2005.

76 Kataoka N, Kuramoto W, Fujiyoshi F: Clinical investigation of professional oral care and pneumonia inflammation for hematopoietic stem cell transplant patients, Journal of Dental Health, 57: 564, 2007.

77 Iwamoto Y, Nishimura F, Soga Y, Takeuchi K, Kurihara M, Takashiba S Murayama Y: Antimicrobial periodontal treatment decrease serum C-reactive protein, tumor necrosis factor-alpha, but not adiponectin, levels in patients with chronic periodontitis, I Periodontal, 74: 1231-1236, 2003.

78 Sonis ST: Mucositis as a biological process: a new hypothesis for the development of chemotherapy-induced stomatotoxicity, Oral Oncology, 34: 39-43, 1998.

79 Yoshida M, Tsubaki K, Kobayashi T, Tanimoto M, Kuriyama K, Murakami H, Minami S, Hiraoka A, Takahashi, Naoe T, Asou N, Kageyama S, Tomonaga M, Saito H, Ohno R: Int Hematol, 70: 261-267, 1999.

80 The Japan Society for Hematopoietic Cell Transplantation : JSHCT Monograph Vol.3, The Japan Society for Hematopoietic Cell Transplantation Web, 14 May, 2007, http://www.jshct.com.

Chapter **6**

Management of Oral Adverse Events

Chapter 6 Management of Oral Adverse Events

The management of oral adverse events is a critical factor influencing prognosis. Oral adverse events include oral mucositis, oral bacterial infections, oral bleeding, graft-versus-host disease (GvHD), dry mouth, and exacerbation of periodontal disease. Various guidelines on the management of these issues have been reported from multiple institutions.

1. Oral Mucositis

Oral mucositis in hematopoietic stem cell transplant (HSCT) patients is a serious condition that can lead to systemic complications and requires appropriate management[1-6]. When oral mucositis develops, proper oral care should be provided based on the severity of the disease and the patient's hematological condition, with a focus on maintaining oral hygiene and alleviating symptoms.

1) Treatment

(1) Oral mucositis can worsen due to local factors, so thorough oral hygiene and local therapy are effective.

(2) Cryotherapy has been studied for patients undergoing high-dose melphalan-containing regimens used in transplants[7,8], but further research is needed.

(3) Gargling with various regimens and management of oral dryness.

(4) Pain control is essential, using gargles containing local anesthetics (such as sodium azulene sulfonate with 4% lidocaine), and for severe pain, opioids like morphine may be administered.

(5) Though reported infrequently, low-level laser therapy has been shown to be effective[9-12], and further research is necessary.

70

2. Oral Bacterial Infections

In HSCT patients, oral mucositis is often accompanied by bacterial infections due to immune dysfunction and reduced salivary gland function. If prolonged severe neutropenia occurs, bacteremia and sepsis caused by oral bacteria can develop[13-16]. During chemotherapy-induced bone marrow suppression, acute infections such as periapical periodontitis and periodontal disease may occur[17-20]. The incidence of oral bacterial infections during chemotherapy has been reported to be 5.8%[21]. Thorough oral care starting before pre-transplant treatment can significantly reduce the risk of these infectious complications[22-24].

Gram-positive bacteria like green streptococci and enterococci are involved in systemic infections with an oral focus. Furthermore, gram-negative bacteria such as Pseudomonas aeruginosa, Neisseria species, and Escherichia coli may also be involved.

Oral bacterial infections can worsen due to local factors, making thorough oral care before the start of transplant treatment essential. Key practices to prevent infections include plaque control using a toothbrush, managing periodontal disease, managing oral dryness, managing oral mucositis, and treating periapical periodontitis. In immunocompromised patients, oral mucositis is often complicated by infections. Severe ulcerative oral mucositis and prolonged neutropenia can lead to dissemination of oral bacteria[13-16]. When neutrophil counts fall below $1,000/mm^3$, the incidence and severity of infections increase[17]. Patients with prolonged neutropenia are at higher risk for severe infections[18, 19]. Moreover, impaired salivary gland function increases the risk of infections with an oral focus. Patients with chronic periodontal disease and reduced bone marrow function may develop systemic infections[21-26].

1) Treatment

(1) Local therapies for periodontal disease include:

Oral care to reduce plaque in neutropenic patients is extremely important.

Local therapies include:

① Gargling with 0.12% chlorhexidine gluconate (not approved in Japan)

② Administering antibiotics (such as minocycline, azithromycin, doxycycline) into periodontal pockets

③ Proper self-care with a toothbrush for plaque control

④ Regular professional mechanical tooth cleaning (PMTC)

3. Oral Candidiasis

Oral candidiasis is caused by opportunistic overgrowth of C. albicans. Several factors contribute to the development of oral candidiasis, such as bone marrow suppression, damage to oral mucosa, and reduced salivary secretion. Additionally, antibiotic use can lead to microbial shifts, increasing the risk of fungal overgrowth[25]. Local antifungal agents like nystatin, amphotericin B gargles, and miconazole gel are commonly used, though their effectiveness in preventing or treating fungal infections in neutropenic patients may vary[26, 27].

1) Treatment

Oral candidiasis is generally caused by opportunistic overgrowth of C. albicans, a normal oral commensal in most individuals. Various factors, including drug- or disease-induced bone marrow dysfunction, oral mucosal damage, impaired salivary gland function, and changes in the oral microbiome due to antibiotic use, contribute to the development of oral candidiasis[25].

(1) Local antifungal agents such as nystatin, amphotericin B gargles, and miconazole gel are commonly used, but their efficacy in preventing or treating fungal infections in

neutropenic patients varies[26, 27].

(2) Local treatments are useful for superficial oral candidiasis, but for persistent fungal infections, systemic fluconazole is often administered, and it has been shown to be effective for preventing and treating oral fungal infections in cancer patients[28].

4. Oral Bleeding

Oral bleeding can occur due to thrombocytopenia and coagulopathy, which increase bleeding tendency as a result of treatment. This is a concern in HSCT patients[22]. Gingival bleeding is more likely to occur when platelet counts fall below 20,000/mm3, especially when gingivitis or periodontitis is already present. Even regular brushing can lead to gingival bleeding when these conditions are present.

In patients with bleeding tendencies, avoiding plaque control by brushing could increase the risk of infection. Additionally, it may lead to plaque accumulation, which heightens the risk of local and systemic infections. Even in patients with bleeding tendencies, regular periodontal evaluations can enable safe plaque control using a toothbrush.

HSCT patients may develop bleeding tendencies due to radiation therapy or chemotherapy, leading to oral bleeding, which can have a significant impact on prognosis if it becomes severe.

1) Treatment

(1) In cases of thrombocytopenia, platelet transfusions may be required in addition to local treatments.

(2) Local treatments for oral bleeding include pressure hemostasis, vasoconstrictors (epinephrine), and hemostatic agents (local thrombin preparations, hemostatic collagen).

Chapter 6 Management of Oral Adverse Events

5. GvHD

Patients undergoing allogeneic HSCT or unrelated donor transplants are at risk of developing graft-versus-host disease (GvHD)[29, 30]. Acute GvHD typically develops 10 to 14 days after transplantation, with mucosal erythema, erosions, ulcers, and blister formation being typical symptoms.

Chronic oral GvHD often resembles autoimmune diseases like lichen planus, pemphigus, and Sjögren's syndrome.

1) Treatment

(1) Acute GvHD is treated with systemic steroids, and local therapies for oral mucosal lesions include steroids and azathioprine gargles[16, 31]. Moisturizing treatments are also essential to protect the mucosa.

(2) Chronic oral GvHD often resembles autoimmune diseases like lichen planus, pemphigus, and Sjögren's syndrome. Oral GvHD is associated with pre-cancerous lesions and malignancies in the oral cavity. Local treatment for chronic GvHD is similar to acute GvHD, with a focus on moisturizing. Moisturizing gel is applied to the buccal mucosa and tongue, and petroleum jelly is applied to the teeth to avoid mechanical irritation of the mucosa.

(3) Other local treatments include steroids and azathioprine gargles. While local cyclosporine has been suggested as beneficial, there are few reliable reports. In Western countries, systemic pilocarpine or cevimeline is considered effective for patients with severe dry mouth, provided that some salivary gland function is preserved. However, these medications are not approved in Japan.

6. Dry Mouth

Dry mouth occurs due to impaired salivary gland function. In HSCT patients, salivary gland dysfunction is common due to pre-transplant conditioning with radiation and chemotherapy, or GvHD[32]. This increases the likelihood of developing dry mouth. The loss of lubrication by saliva can lead to mucosal damage, while decreased self-cleansing ability results in plaque accumulation, and impaired salivary buffering capacity increases the risk of caries. The pathogenicity of the oral microbiome may also increase. Therefore, early oral care is critical. Local treatments with various artificial saliva or saliva substitutes, as well as moisturizers, are effective. Systemic administration of pilocarpine or cevimeline is considered effective, but they are not approved in Japan.

1) Treatment

Dry mouth is commonly observed in HSCT patients. Impaired salivary gland function increases the risk of caries and periodontal disease and makes the development of oral mucositis more likely, raising the risk of infections from mucositis. Moreover, GvHD-related mucositis can worsen, making the prevention and treatment of dry mouth crucial.

(1) Treatment for dry mouth includes local use of various artificial saliva substitutes or moisturizers, as well as mouth rinses, moisturizing gels, and sprays. The frequency of moisturizer use is reported to range from a few times a day to around 10 times a day. Gels tend to have a longer-lasting moisturizing effect, but if oral mucositis is severe, they may be difficult to apply, so gargles or sprays may be used in combination.

(Hitoshi Osano, Department of Dentistry and Oral and Maxillofacial Surgery, Jichi Medical University Saitama Medical Center)

References

1 Elting LS, Cooksley C, Chambers M, et al: The burdens of cancer therapy. Clinical and economic outcomes of chemotherapy-induced mucositis, Cancer, 98 (7): 1531-1539, 2003.

2 Elting LS, Cooksley CD, Chambers MS, et al: Risk, outcomes, and costs of radiation-induced oral mucositis among patients with head-and-neck malignancies, Int J Radiat Oncol Biol Phys, 68 (4): 1110-1120, 2007.

3 Lalla RV, Sonis ST, Peterson DE: Management of oral mucositis in patients who have cancer, Dent Clin North Am, 52 (1): 61-77, viii, 2008.

4 Peterson DE, Lalla RV: Oral mucositis: The new paradigms, Curr Opin Oncol, 22 (4): 318-322, 2010.

5 Rosenthal DI: Consequences of mucositis-induced treatment breaks and dose reductions on head and neck cancer treatment outcomes, J Support Oncol, 5 (9 Suppl 4): 23-31, 2007.

6 Sonis ST, Oster G, Fuchs H, et al: Oral mucositis and the clinical and economic outcomes of hematopoietic stem-cell transplantation, J Clin Oncol, 19 (8): 2201-2205, 2001.

7 Rocke LK, Loprinzi CL, Lee JK, et al: A randomized clinical trial of two different durations of oral cryotherapy for prevention of 5-fluorouracil-related stomatitis, Cancer, 72 (7): 2234-2238, 1993.

8 Mori T, Yamazaki R, Aisa Y, et al: Brief oral cryotherapy for the prevention of high-dose melphalan-induced stomatitis in allogeneic hematopoietic stem cell transplant recipients, Support Care Cancer, 14 (4): 392-395, 2006.

9 Spielberger R, Stiff P, Bensinger W, et al: Palifermin for oral mucositis after intensive therapy for hematologic cancers, N Engl J Med, 351(25): 2590-2598, 2004.

10 Rosen LS, Abdi E, Davis ID, et al: Palifermin reduces the incidence of oral mucositis in patients with metastatic colorectal cancer treated with fluorouracil-basedchemotherapy, J Clin Oncol, 24(33): 5194-5200, 2006.

11 Antunes HS, de Azevedo AM, da Silva Bouzas LF, Adão CA, Pinheiro CT, Mayhe R, Pinheiro LH, Azevedo R, Matos VD, Rodrigues PC, Small IA, Zangaro RA, Ferreira CG: Low-power laser in the prevention of induced oral mucositis in bone marrow transplantation patients: a randomized trial, Blood, 109(5): 2250-2255, 2007.

12 Chor A, Torres SR, Maiolino A, Nucci M: Low-power laser to prevent oral mucositis in autologous hematopoietic stem cell transplantation, Eur, J Haematol, 84(2): 178-179, 2010.

13 Lalla RV, Brennan MT, Schubert MM: Oral complications of cancer therapy Pharmacology and Therapeutics for Dentistry, 6th ed, Mo Mosby Elsevier, St. Louis, 782-798, 2011.

14 Schubert MM, Peterson DE: Oral complications of hematopoietic cell transplantation Thomas' Hematopoietic Cell Transplantation Stem Cell Transplantation, 4th ed, Wiley-Blackwell, Oxford UK, 1589-1607, 2009.

15 De Pauw BE, Donnelly JP: Infections in the immunocompromised host: general principles, Mandell, Douglas, and Bennett's Principles and Practices of Infectious Diseases, 5th ed, Churchill Livingstone, Philadelphia Pa, 3079-3090, 2000.

16 Kennedy HF, Morrison D, Kaufmann ME, et al: Origins of Staphylococcus epidermidis and Streptococcus oralis causing bacteraemia in a bone marrow transplant patient, J Med Microbiol, 49 (4): 367-370, 2000.

17 Rolston KVI, Bodey GP: Infections in patients with cancer Holland-Frei Cancer Medicine, 8th ed, People's Medical Publishing House-USA, Shelton, 1921-1940, 2010.

18 Giamarellou H, Antoniadou A: Infectious complications of febrile leukopenia, Infect Dis Clin North Am, 15 (2): 457-482, 2001.

19 Zambelli A, Montagna D, Da Prada GA, et al: Evaluation of infectious complications and immune recovery following high-dose chemotherapy (HDC) and autologous peripheral blood progenitor cell transplantation (PBPC-T) in 148 breast cancer patients, Anticancer Res, 22 (6B): 3701-3708, 2002.

20 Schubert MM, Peterson DE: Oral complications of hematopoietic cell transplantation. Thomas' Hematopoietic Cell Transplantation: Stem Cell Transplantation, 4th ed, Wiley-Blackwell, Oxford UK, 1589-1607, 2009.

21 Peterson DE, Minah GE, Overholser CD, et al: Microbiology of acute periodontal infection in myelosuppressed cancer patients, J Clin Oncol, 5 (9): 1461-1468, 1987.

22 Graber CJ, de Almeida KN, Atkinson JC, et al: Dental health and viridans streptococcal bacteremia in allogeneic hematopoietic stem cell transplant recipients, Bone Marrow Transplant, 27 (5): 537-542, 2001.

Chapter 6 Management of Oral Adverse Events

23 Akintoye SO, Brennan MT, Graber CJ, et al: A retrospective investigation of advanced periodontal disease as a risk factor for septicemia in hematopoietic stem cell and bone marrow transplant recipients, Oral Surg Oral Med Oral Pathol Oral Radiol Endod, 94 (5): 581-588, 2002.

24 Raber-Durlacher JE, Epstein JB, Raber J, et al: Periodontal infection in cancer patients treated with high-dose chemotherapy, Support Care Cancer, 10 (6): 466-473, 2002.

25 Böhme A, Karthaus M, Hoelzer D: Antifungal prophylaxis in neutropenic patients with hematologic malignancies, Antibiot Chemother, 50: 69-78, 2000.

26 Epstein JB, Vickars L, Spinelli J, et al: Efficacy of chlorhexidine and nystatin rinses in prevention of oral complications in leukemia and bone marrow transplantation, Oral Surg Oral Med Oral Pathol, 73 (6): 682-689, 1992.

27 Ellis ME, Clink H, Ernst P, et al: Controlled study of fluconazole in the prevention of fungal infections in neutropenic patients with haematological malignancies and bone marrow transplant recipients, Eur J Clin Microbiol Infect Dis, 13 (1): 3-11, 1994.

28 Lalla RV, Latortue MC, Hong CH, et al: A systematic review of oral fungal infections in patients receiving cancer therapy, Support Care Cancer, 18 (8): 985-992, 2010.

29 Schubert MM, Peterson DE: Oral complications of hematopoietic cell transplantation, Thomas' Hematopoietic Cell Transplantation Stem Cell Transplantation, 4th ed, Wiley-Blackwell, Oxford UK, 1589-1607, 2009.

30 Demarosi F, Bez C, Sardella A. et al: Oral involvement in chronic graft-vs-host disease following allogenic bone marrow transplantation, Arch Dermatol, 138(6): 842-843, 2002.

31 Epstein JB, Nantel S, Sheoltch SM: Topical azathioprine in the combined treatment of chronic oral graft-versus-host disease, Bone Marrow Transplant, 25(6): 683-687, 2000.

32 Jensen SB, Pederson AM, Vissink A, et al: A systematic review of salivary gland hypofunction and xerostomia induced by cancer therapies: prevalence, severity and impact on quality of life, Support Care Cancer, 18(8): 1039-1060, 2010.

Chapter 7

Follow-up Observation

Chapter 7 Follow-up Observation

Hematopoietic stem cell transplant (HSCT) patients require long-term management of complications even after graft engraftment, as immune function takes time to recover. Common late oral complications following HSCT include dry mouth due to reduced salivary gland function, GvHD, and secondary malignant tumors in the oral cavity. Furthermore, leukemia or lymphoma patients may experience recurrence of their disease in the oral cavity. For these reasons, long-term follow-up observation of the oral cavity is necessary.

1. The Need for Follow-up Observation in Managing Oral Adverse Events

Few studies have discussed whether follow-up observation of the oral cavity contributes to the treatment outcomes of HSCT patients. However, the management of adverse events after HSCT is important[1,2], and long-term management of oral adverse events is recommended.

Oral complications after HSCT include: 1) Infection prevention until immune function recovers, 2) GvHD, 3) Secondary cancers in the oral cavity, 4) Recurrence of the underlying disease, 5) Salivary gland dysfunction, 6) dysgeusia.

1) Infection Prevention

Thorough plaque control until immune function recovers after transplantation is essential for reducing the incidence and severity of oral complications caused by malignancy treatments[2-5]. In addition to the expected side effects of chemotherapy and radiation therapy, it is necessary to provide a theoretical basis for the importance of maintaining oral hygiene. Thorough oral hygiene is crucial at all stages of treatment, starting from before cancer treatment.

80

2) Oral GvHD

In patients with chronic GvHD, where there is immune dysfunction, it is recommended to avoid dental treatment for one year after immune transplantation unless there is an emergency[6]. GvHD is recognized as a complication that affects the outcomes of allogeneic transplantation[7-13]. GvHD can affect the oral mucosa and is considered a risk factor for oral cancer, so its management is important. Long-term monitoring is necessary, as GvHD can persist for extended periods. According to the Japan Society for Hematopoietic Stem Cell Transplantation guidelines[14], chronic oral GvHD is characterized by mucosal lichen planus-like lesions, leukoplakia (excessive keratinization), and sclerotic changes in the mouth and surrounding skin. As leukoplakia needs to be differentiated from secondary cancer (squamous cell carcinoma), regular biopsies are recommended.

3) Secondary Cancer in the Oral Cavity

Soft tissue tumors and lymphadenopathy observed in post-transplant patients are considered to potentially represent secondary primary malignancies such as lymphoproliferative disorders.

4) Recurrence of the Primary Disease

Leukemia and malignant lymphoma may infiltrate the oral cavity[15-26]. Gum infiltration, oral infections, and bleeding may indicate disease recurrence, especially in patients being treated for leukemia or lymphoma.

5) Salivary Gland Dysfunction and Dysgeusia

Chemotherapy and radiation therapy before transplantation can lead to salivary gland dysfunction, increasing the risk of periodontal disease and dental caries. Continuous plaque control is necessary. Furthermore, dysgeusia can lead to decreased appetite, so ongoing management is required.

Chapter 7 Follow-up Observation

2. Follow-up Interval and Duration After Hematopoietic Stem Cell Transplantation

1) There are few studies on the intervals and duration of follow-up for oral complications. According to United States guidelines[27], if the patient's condition is stable, it is recommended to follow up once a week for the first month after discharge, then every two weeks for the next two months, and once a month thereafter until two months after discharge.

2) Secondary cancers are known to develop after transplantation, including squamous cell carcinoma in the oral cavity[28-47]. According to Kruse[37], the most common onset of oral cancer occurs 5 to 9 years after transplantation, with a strong correlation to chronic GvHD. Therefore, for patients with chronic GvHD in the oral cavity, stringent observation is recommended even after the fifth year.

(Hitoshi Osano, Department of Dentistry and Oral and Maxillofacial Surgery, Jichi Medical University Saitama Medical Center)

References

1 Flowers MED, Deeg HJ: Delayed complications after hematopoietic cell transplantation, Thoms' Hematopoietic cell Transplantation, Third edition, Wiley-Blackwell, Malden,MA, 944-961, 2004.

2 Akintoye SO, Brennan MT, Graber CJ, McKinney BE, Rams TE, Barrett AJ, et al: A retrospective investigation of advanced periodontal disease as a risk factor for septicemia in hematopoietic stem cell and bone marrow transplant recipients, Oral Surg Oral Med Oral Pathol Oral Radiol Endod, 94(5): 581-588, 2002.

3 Dobr T, Passweg J, Weber C, Tichelli A, Heim D, Meyer J, et al: Oral health risks associated with HLA-types of patients undergoing hematopoietic stem cell transplantation, Eur J Haematol, 78(6): 495-499, 2007.

4 Soga Y, Saito T, Nishimura F, Ishimaru F, Mineshiba J, Mineshiba F, et al: Appearance of multidrug-resistant opportunistic bacteria on the gingiva during leukemia treatment, J Periodontol, 79(1): 181-186, 2008.

5 Soga Y, Yamasuji Y, Kudo C, Matsuura-Yoshimoto K, Yamabe K, Sugiura Y, et al: Febrile neutropenia and periodontitis: lessons from a case periodontal treatment in the intervals between chemotherapy cycles for leukemia reduced febrile neutropenia, Support Care Cancer, 17(5): 581-587, 2009.

6 Demarosi F, Lodi G, Carrassi A, Moneghini L, Sarina B, Sardella A: Clinical and histopathological features of the oral mucosa in allogeneic haematopoietic stem cell transplantation patients, Exp Oncol, 29(4): 304-308, 2007.

7 Reyes AD, Martín TA, Leache EB, Suárez EC: Oral manifestations of graft versus host disease. Case report, Med Oral, 8(5): 361-365, 2003.

8 Jaźwińska AG, Kozak I, Prystupiuk EK, Rokicka M, Ganowicz E, Trojaczek JD, et al: Transient oral cavity and skin complications after mucositis preventing therapy (palifermin) in a patient after allogeneic PBSCT, Case history, Adv Med Sci, 51 (Suppl 1): 66-68, 2006.

9 Imanguli MM, Alevizos I, Brown R, Pavletic SZ, Atkinson JC: Oral graft-versus-host disease. Oral Dis, 14(5):396-412, 2008.

Chapter 7 Follow-up Observation

10 Khan FM, Sy S, Louie P, Ugarte-Torres A, Berka N, Sinclair GD, et al: Genomic instability after allogeneic hematopoietic cell transplantation is frequent in oral mucosa, particularly in patients with a history of chronic graft-versus-host disease, and rare in nasal mucosa, Blood, 116(10): 1803-1806, 2010.

11 Treister NS, Cook EF, Antin J, Lee SJ, Soiffer R, Woo SB: Clinical evaluation of oral chronic graft-versus-host disease, Biol Blood Marrow Transplant, 14(1): 110-115, 2008.

12 Treister NS, Woo SB, O'Holleran EW, Lehmann LE, Parsons SK, Guinan EC: Oral chronic graft-versus-host disease in pediatric patients after hematopoietic stem cell transplantation, Biol Blood Marrow Transplant, 11(9): 721-731, 2005.

13 Ahmad I, Labbé AC, Chagnon M, Busque L, Cohen S, Kiss T, et al: Incidence and prognostic value of eosinophilia in chronic graft-versus host disease after nonmyeloablative hematopoietic cell transplantation, Biol Blood Marrow Transplant, 17(11): 1673-1678, 2011.

14 Apanese Society for Hematopoietic Cell Transplantation: Hematopoietic Cell Transplantation Guidelines-GVHD, Guidelines of the Japanese Society for Hematology, 2008.

15 Allabert C, Estève E, Joly P, Troussard X, Comoz F, Courville P, et al: Mucosal involvement in lymphomatoid papulosis: four cases, Ann Dermatol Venereol, 135(4): 273-278, 2008.

16 Cabane J, Godeau P, Chomette G, Auriol M, Szpirglass H, Raphael M: Buccal lymphomatoid granulomatosis, Rev Med Interne, 11(1): 69-72, 1990.

17 Chimenti S, Fargnoli MC, Pacifico A, Peris K: Mucosal involvement in a patient with lymphomatoid papulosis, J Am Acad Dermatol, 44(2 Suppl): 339-341, 2001.

18 Río Ed, Yus ES, Requena L, Puente LG, Veiga HV: Oral pseudolymphoma: a report of two cases, J Cutan Pathol, 24(1): 51-55, 1997.

19 Bschorer R, Lingenfelser T, Kaiserling E, Schwenzer N: Malignant lymphoma of the mucosa-associated lymphoid tissue (MALT)--consecutive unusual manifestation in the rectum and gingiva, J Oral Pathol Med, 22(4): 190-192, 1993.

20 Dodd CL, Greenspan D, Heinic GS, Rabanus JP, Greenspan JS: Multi-focal oral non-Hodgkin's lymphoma in an AIDS patient, Br Dent J, 175(10): 373-377, 1993.

21 Atkinson K, Biggs J, Concannon A, Dodds A, Dale B, Norman J: Second marrow transplants for

84

recurrence of haematological malignancy, Bone Marrow Transplant, 1(2): 159-166, 1986.

22 Haznedaroğlu IC, Ustündağ Y, Benekli M, Savaş MC, Safali M, Dündar SV: Isolated gingival relapse during complete hematological remission in acute promyelocytic leukemia, Acta Haematol, 93(1): 54-55, 1995.

23 Izumi T, Hatake K, Imagawa S, Yoshikda M, Ohta M, Sasaki R, et al: A case of acute promyelocytic leukemia (APL) with myeloblastoma in the oral cavity developing after receiving all-trans retinoic acid (ATRA), Rinsho Ketsueki, 35(6): 598-602, 1994.

24 Maygarden SJ, Askin FB, Burkes EJ, McMillan C, Sanders JE: Isolated extramedullary relapse of acute myelogenous leukemia in a tooth, Mod Pathol, 2(1): 59-62, 1989.

25 Papamanthos MK, Kolokotronis AE, Skulakis HE, Fericean AM, Zorba MT, Matiakis AT: Acute myeloid leukaemia diagnosed by intra-oral myeloid sarcoma. A case report, Head Neck Pathol, 4(2): 132-135, 2010.

26 Yoo SW, Chung EJ, Kim SY, Ko JH, Baek HS, Lee HJ, et al: Multiple extramedullary relapses without bone marrow involvement after second allogeneic hematopoietic stem cell transplantation for acute myeloid leukemia, Pediatr Transplant, 16(4): E125-129, 2012.

27 Fred Hutchinson Cancer Research Center, Seattle Cancer Care Alliance: Long-Term Follow-Up After Hematopoietic Stem Cell Transplant Eneral Guidelines for Referring Physicians, Version April 2011.

28 Arai Y, Arai H, Aoyagi A, Yamagata T, Mitani K, Kubota K, et al: A solid tumor of donor cell-origin after allogeneic peripheral blood stem cell transplantation, Am J Transplant, 6(12): 3042-3043, 2006.

29 Au WY, Chan EC, Pang A, Lie AK, Liang R, Yuen AP, et al: Nonhematologic malignancies after allogeneic hematopoietic stem cell transplantation: incidence and molecular monitoring, Bone Marrow Transplant, 34(11): 981-985, 2004.

30 Ben-Yosef R, Braverman I, Saah D, Nagler R, Shohat S, Or R, et al: Mucosal melanoma following autologous stem cell transplantation for non-Hodgkin's lymphoma (NHL), Bone Marrow Transplant, 18(5): 1017-1019, 1996.

31 Demarosi F, Lodi G, Carrassi A, Soligo D, Sardella A: Oral malignancies following HSCT: graft versus host disease and other risk factors, Oral Oncol, 41(9): 865-877, 2005.

Chapter 7 Follow-up Observation

32 Elad S, Levitt M, MY S: Chronic graft-versus-host-disease involving the oral mucosa: clinical presentation and treatment, Refuat Hapeh Vehashinayim, 25(4): 19-27, 72, 2008.

33 Fujii H, Ueda Y, Nakagawa H: Secondary solid tumors in autologous-peripheral blood stem cell transplantation recipients, Rinsho Ketsueki, 41(8): 621-627, 2000.

34 Hamadah I, Binamer Y, Alajlan S, Nassar A, Saleh AJ: Squamous cell carcinoma of the lip after allogeneic hemopoietic stem cell transplantation, Hematol Oncol Stem Cell Ther, 3(2): 84-88, 2010.

35 Keating MJ: Chronic lymphocytic leukemia. Clinical oral poster session, Hematol Cell Ther, 42(1): 35-39, 2000.

36 Khan FM, Sy S, Louie P, Ugarte-Torres A, Berka N, Sinclair GD, et al: Genomic instability after allogeneic hematopoietic cell transplantation is frequent in oral mucosa, particularly in patients with a history of chronic graft-versus-host disease, and rare in nasal mucosa, Blood, 116(10): 1803-1806, 2010.

37 Kruse AL, Grätz KW: Oral carcinoma after hematopoietic stem cell transplantation-a new classification based on a literature review over 30 years, Head Neck Oncol, 1: 29, 2009.

38 Lee SJ, Flowers ME: Recognizing and managing chronic graft-versus-host disease, Hematology Am Soc Hematol Educ Program, 134-141, 2008.

39 Majhail NS, Brazauskas R, Rizzo JD, Sobecks RM, Wang Z, Horowitz MM, et al: Secondary solid cancers after allogeneic hematopoietic cell transplantation using busulfan-cyclophosphamide conditioning, Blood, 117(1): 316-322, 2011.

40 Meier JK, Wolff D, Pavletic S, Greinix H, Gosau M, Bertz H, et al: Oral chronic graft-versus-host disease: report from the International Consensus Conference on clinical practice in cGVHD, Clin Oral Investig, 15(2): 127-139, 2011.

41 Munakata W, Sawada T, Kobayashi T, Kakihana K, Yamashita T, Ohashi K, et al: Mortality and medical morbidity beyond 2 years after allogeneic hematopoietic stem cell transplantation: experience at a single institution, Int J Hematol, 93(4): 517-522, 2011.

42 Noguchi K, Nakase M, Inui M, Nakamura S, Okumura K, Tagawa T: A case of tongue carcinoma associated with chronic graft-versus-host disease after allogeneic haematopoietic stem cell transplantation, Aust Dent J, 55(2): 200-202, 2010.

43 Petropoulos D, Worth LL, Mullen CA, Madden R, Mahajan A, Choroszy M, et al: Total body irradiation, fludarabine, melphalan, and allogeneic hematopoietic stem cell transplantation for advanced pediatric hematologic malignancies, Bone Marrow Transplant, 37(5): 463-467, 2006.

44 Reddy NM, Sullivan MA, Hahn TE, Battiwalla M, Smiley SL, McCarthy PL: Association of squamous cell carcinoma of the oral cavity in allogeneic hematopoietic stem cell transplant recipients, Bone Marrow Transplant, 40(9): 907-909, 2007.

45 Resende RG, Correia-Silva JeF, Galvão CF, Gomes CC, Carneiro MA, Gomez RS: Oral leukoplakia in a patient with Fanconi anemia: recurrence or a new primary lesion?, J Oral Maxillofac Surg, 69(7): 1940-1943, 2011.

46 Szeto CH, Shek TW, Lie AK, Au WY, Yuen AP, Kwong YL: Squamous cell carcinoma of the tongue complicating chronic oral mucosal graft-versus-host disease after allogeneic hematopoietic stem cell transplantation, Am J Hematol, 77(2): 200-202, 2004.

47 Woo HJ, Bai CH, Kim YD, Song SY: Mucoepidermoid carcinoma of the submandibular gland after chemotherapy in a child, Auris Nasus Larynx, 36(2): 244-246, 2009.

Chapter **8**

Prevention and Treatment in Children

Chapter 8 Prevention and Treatment in Children

1. Characteristics of Hematopoietic Stem Cell Transplantation in Children

With advances in multidisciplinary treatment, the treatment outcomes for pediatric hematologic and oncological diseases have improved, achieving treatment rates of over 70%[1]. The results of allogeneic stem cell transplantation (allo-SCT) for refractory cases now show long-term survival rates of over 60%[2]. While allo-SCT plays a major role in treating refractory diseases, various issues in long-term survivors of transplantation have become apparent[3], requiring appropriate management.

In children, who are still in a stage of growth, the impact of transplantation on growth cannot be overlooked, unlike in adults, who are fully developed individuals. If transplantation occurs before the eruption of permanent teeth, the effects on the teeth can be significant[4]. This section focuses on late post-transplant complications related to the teeth and discusses issues unique to children.

2. Oral Adverse Events in Children

Oral adverse events that occur during hematopoietic stem cell transplantation and its preconditioning, such as dry mouth, mucositis, neuropathy, and increased susceptibility to infections, are the same in children as they are in adults, and the evaluation and management are similar to those for adults.

As late post-transplant complications, not only issues common to adults, such as secondary cancers, but also problems specific to children in the growth phase may arise, including abnormalities in the teeth and disturbances in jaw growth[4-7].

＊ Tooth Abnormalities Based on the Timing of Transplantation:

· Period before crown formation: formation defects such as missing teeth or microdontia.

· Period before root formation: abnormalities in root morphology, such as short roots.

Table 6 shows the developmental stages of permanent teeth[8].

Table 6 Development of permanent teeth

Type of tooth	Tooth germ formation	Initial calcification	Crown completed	Eruption	Root completed
First molar	3.5-4 mo I.U.	at birth	2.5-4 yr	6-7 yr	9-10 yr
Central incisor	5 mo I.U.	3-4 mo	4-5 yr	6-8 yr	9-10 yr
Lateral incisor	5.5 mo I.U.	3-4 mk	4-5 yr	7-9 yr	10-11 yr
Canine	5.5-6 mo I.U.	4-5 mo	6-7 yr	9-12 yr	12-15 yr
First premolar	at birth	1.5-2 yr	5-6 yr	10-12 yr	12-13 yr
Second premolar	7.5-8 mo	2-2.5 yr	6-7 yr	10-12 yr	12-14 yr
Second molar	8.5-9 mo	2.5-3 yr	7-8 yr	10-13 yr	14-16 yr
Third molar	3.5-4 yr	7-10 yr	12-16 yr	17-21 yr	18-25 yr

Abbreviations: 1.U. = in utero, wk = weeks, mo = months, yr = years.

Due to developmental defects in permanent teeth and reduced jaw growth, early tooth loss, occlusal abnormalities, and an increased risk of dental caries and periodontal disease may occur. Therefore, panoramic X-rays should be used for a comprehensive evaluation, and long-term follow-up, including oral care, is necessary to ensure early detection of caries and periodontal disease and to restore oral function.

Chapter 8 Prevention and Treatment in Children

3. Considerations and Precautions for Oral Examination in Children

Unlike adults, children may be unwilling to cooperate due to fear, even if they understand the need for treatment. It can be particularly difficult to conduct an oral examination after symptoms have developed. Therefore, it is crucial to assess the condition of the oral cavity before treatment starts, build trust, and focus on prevention as much as possible.

Additionally, obtaining the understanding of parents is very important, and thorough explanations are necessary, not only about oral care and treatment but also regarding the potential for late complications.

4. Key Points for Oral Care Nursing in Children

1) Factors that influence oral care in children include the child's age, cognitive level, understanding of the disease, overall health status, presence of a caregiver, and daily living habits[9,10].

2) Instruction on proper brushing techniques should be provided based on the child's age and cognitive ability.

3) During hospitalization, it is important to understand the child's daily habits and improve their awareness of tooth brushing and oral hygiene to prevent mucositis and dry mouth.

4) Nursing care for oral hygiene based on developmental stages[11,12]:

92

(1) Infant: Explain the importance of establishing a tooth brushing routine to parents and raise their awareness to ensure they can care for the child with a stable mindset.

(2) Early Childhood: Clearly express and explain the importance of establishing a tooth brushing habit to the child. Engage in preparatory activities through pretend play or acceptance play, helping the child to become familiar with the process.

(3) Late Childhood: Support the child in understanding and continuing the habit of brushing their teeth. Use visual media such as "picture books," "photos," or "dolls" to identify the child's communication preferences and proceed with the method that works best for them.

(4) School Age: Continue to reinforce oral cleaning and cavity prevention, and maintain brushing habits. Written communication is possible at this stage, and preparation techniques can be utilized to make the process easier for the child.

(5) Adolescence: Maintaining oral cleanliness and preventing cavities remains crucial during this period.

5) Provide families with knowledge about mucositis and oral care methods, encouraging the child to develop these habits independently. However, it is important to consider the family's needs and ensure that they do not become overwhelmed by the care responsibilities.

(Masahide Mizutani, Department of Oral and Maxillofacial Surgery, Osaka Women's and Children's Hospital,

Tomoko Fukuchi, 4th Floor West Ward, Osaka Women's and Children's Hospital,

Masami Inoue, Department of Hematology/Oncology, Osaka Women's and Children's Hospital)

References

1 Sawada A, Kawa T: Progress in the treatment of childhood cancer, Pediatrics, 46: 1933-1940, 2005.

2 Japanese Society for Hematopoietic Cell Transplantation: 2007 National Survey Report, Japanese Society for Hematopoietic Cell Transplantation Data Center, Nagoya, 2008.

3 Ishida Y: Late complications after hematopoietic stem cell transplantation for childhood cancer, Journal of the Japanese Academy of Pediatrics, 112: 1505-1518, 2008.

4 Holtta P, et al: Agenesis and microdontia of permanent teeth as late adverse effects after stem cell transplantation in young children, Cancer, 103: 181-190, 2005.

5 Voskuilen IGM, Veerkamp JSJ, et al: Long-term adverse effects of hematopoietic stem cell transplantation on dental development in children, Support Care Cancer, 17: 1169-1175, 2009.

6 Vaughan MD, et al: Dental abnormalities in children preparing for pediatric bone marrow transplantation, Bone marrow transplant, 36: 863-866, 2004.

7 Miho Y, Ikeda S, et al: Disorders of tooth formation observed after hematopoietic stem cell transplantation therapy in children-Comparison of leukemia, neuroblastoma and severe aplastic anemia-Journal of the Society of Dentistry for the Disabled, 30: 29-38, 2009.

8 Original author by Fujita K, revised by Kirino C: Anatomy of teeth, 21st edition, Kanehara Publishing, Tokyo, 124, 1989.

9 Muramatsu M: Learning oral care for various patients from the basics, Nursing Today, 24: 18-51, 2009.

10 Toyoshima M, Sako Y, et al: Oral care for children undergoing chemotherapy - Study on the introduction of brushing (bath method) , Journal of Osaka Prefectural Maternal and Child Health Medical Center, 22: 48-52, 2006.

11 Tanaka K: Preparation guidebook that can be used in pediatric medical settings - Knowledge and points for fun and effective implementation - "Chapter 3: Understanding cognitive development and disease - What is preparation?" 1st edition, Nissoken, Nagoya, 31-35, 2003.

12 Thomson RH, Stanford G: Child life in hospitals: A "play" program that supports children's minds. "Chapter 2: Children's reactions to hospitalization." First edition, Chuo Hoki, Tokyo, 19-48, 2003.

MEMO

Materials

Materials: Anatomy and Terminology Necessary for Oral and Dental Evaluation

1. Names of facial parts

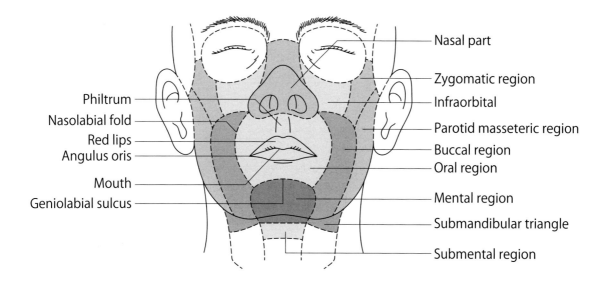

2. Structure of the oral cavity

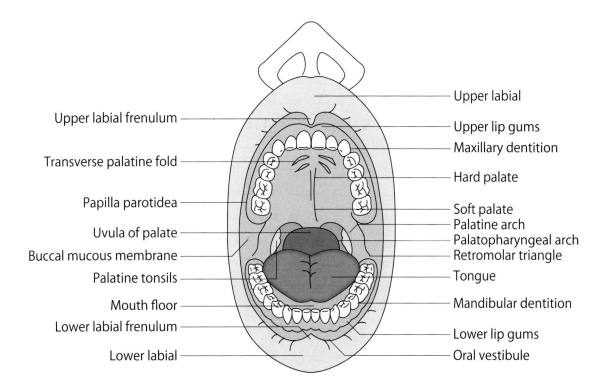

Materials

3. Tooth structure

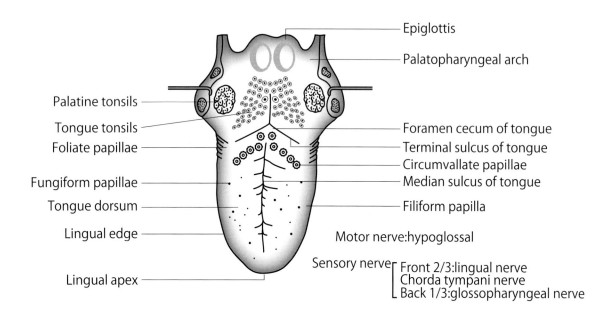

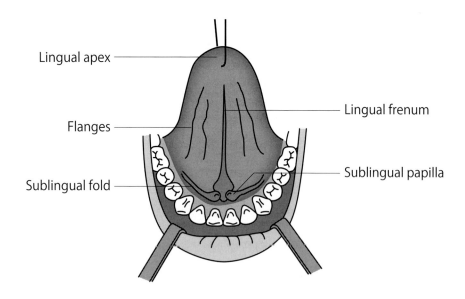

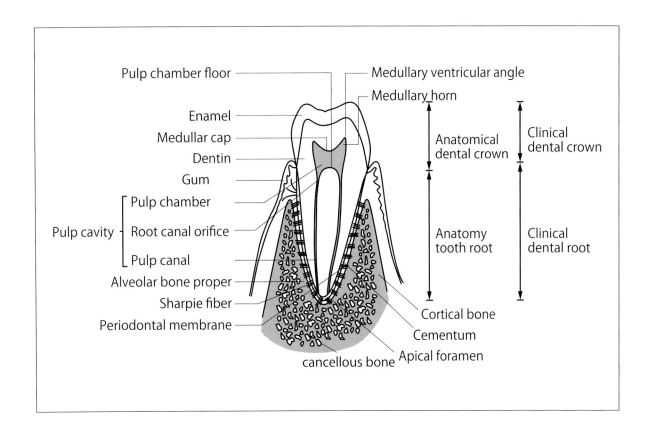

Index

acute GvHD   74

after engraftment   9

allogeneic hematopoietic stem
cell transplantation (allogeneic
transplants)   7

apical periodontitis   56

autologous hematopoietic stem
cell transplantation (autologous
transplants)   7

background   46

bacteremia   60

brushing instruction   50

brushing method   50

caries   56

cevimeline   74

chlorhexidine   52

chronic GvHD   10

chronic oral GvHD   81

clinical guidelines   45

Common Terminology Criteria for
Adverse Events v4.0 Japanese JCOG
version   20

continuous oral care   47

cryotherapy   59, 70

cyclosporin(CSP)   34

dental treatment   54

effectiveness of oral care   48

Eiler J.   17

extraction of wisdom teeth   55

febrile neutropenia   8

gingival bleeding   73

graft-versus-host disease   10

graft-versus-tumor effect   11

HLA   6

human leukocyte antigen   6

leukoplakia   81

lichen planus   81

local treatment for oral bleeding   73

long-term management   80

low-level laser therapy   70

lymphoproliferative disorders   81

marginal periodontitis   57

MASCC   44

methotrexate   10

microdontia   91

moisturizer   51

mouth rinsing   52

myeloablative conditioning   7

oral adverse events   70

oral assessment index   19

oral candidiasis   72

oral care   2

oral mucositis   70

pilocarpine   74

plaque control   50

povidone-iodine   53

preconditioning   90

prevention   46

pulpitis   54

recommended   46

regimen-related toxicity   8

removal of infection sources   56

saline   53

secondary cancer   37

sepsis   60

sodium azulene sulfonate   53

sponge brush   50

standard conditioning   32

systemic adverse events   60

tacrorimus(TAC)   34

Author

The Japanese Society of Oral Care Academic Committee

Akira Arasaki	Izumi Mataga	Yoshiya Ueyama
Akihide Negishi	Setsuko Itoh	Yoshiaki Shimizu
Kazuto Hoshi	Kazumi Koganesawa	Yoshitaka Toyama
Nagato Natsume	Masashi Tatematsu	Masumi Muramatsu
Ryohei Adachi	Hiyori Makino	Masahiro Umeda
Kenji Kawano	Keiko Inoue	Teruyo Shintani
Hajime Sunakawa	Hideo Sakaguchi	Kayoko Nakamura
Makoto Noguchi	Akira Tanaka	Nobuo Motegi
Fusako Kawano	Mitsuyoshi Matsuda	Tetsuro Onishi
Norio Takagi	Hiroshi Imai	Toshio Suzuki
Tetsuo Hanagata	Hideaki Sakashita	Shigetaka Yanagisawa
Hiromitsu Kishimoto	Yutaka Tsutsumi	Susumu Oshimura
Tsuyoshi Takado	Seibun Mikuni	Noriko Suzuki
Daisuke Hinode	Hideto Imura	Morimasa Yamada
Hiroki Iga	Michio Shikimori	Yoshiaki Kamikawa
Keika Gen	Kayo Teraoka	
Yuuki Takeuchi	Masaru Miyata	